We dedicate this book with profound gratitude to all of the physicians who enthusiastically agreed to be interviewed. We are honored by their trust. We are moved by their passion and commitment to healing. Our heartfelt thank you.

The Soul Of The Physician

Doctors Speaking About Passion, Resilience, and Hope

Linda G. Henry and James D. Henry

The Soul of the Physician:
Doctors Speaking About Passion, Resilience, and Hope

Internet address: www.ama-assn.org

This book is for informational purposes only. It is not intended to constitute legal or financial advice. If legal, financial, or other professional advice is required, the services of a competent professional should be sought.

Additional copies of this book may be ordered by calling 800 621-8335.
Secure on-line orders can be taken at www.ama-assn.org/catalog.
Mention product number OP209701.

ISBN 1-57947-244-3
BP37:0099-01:10/01

Linda G. Henry. Linda is the owner and president of Marketing and Communication Strategies, Puyallup, Washington. She is a marketing consultant, specializing in health care, with a special interest in working with organizations experiencing transition. She has more than 16 years of extensive health care marketing experience within for-profit and not-for-profit organizations in diverse settings. Linda has served as director of marketing for both small and large hospitals and an academic medical center. As a consultant, she works with hospitals, hospital corporations, medical practices, and individual physicians and dentists. She is an experienced speaker and conducts seminars on a wide range of business topics, including improving patient–customer satisfaction, communication, and health care issues. Linda is a published author and writes regularly on marketing and business communication issues.

James D. Henry. Jim is principal of Positive Strategies Unlimited, Puyallup, Washington. He has more than 25 years experience in organizational enhancement, management training, and career development. For 10 years he was corporate training manager in Dallas for Texas Utilities, a Fortune 500 company and one of the largest utilities in the nation. Most recently he served as a career-planning consultant for Washington Mutual Bank in Seattle. Jim's consulting business specializes in strategies for enhancing soul in business. As a consultant, he provides customized training programs and vocational consulting services to groups and individuals. An experienced trainer, he facilitates workshops and seminars on such topics as Leading With Soul—Retaining Employees, Managing Your Career, Team Building, and Connecting with the Joy of Medicine. Jim is a published author, writing regularly on business and vocational issues.

Both Linda and Jim are passionate about enhancing soul within health care. They are the authors of *Reclaiming Soul In Health Care, Practical Strategies for Revitalizing Providers of Care,* published in 1999 by the American Hospital Association Press.

CONTENTS

PROLOGUE

We experienced mixed reactions when the American Medical Association (AMA) contacted us about the possibility of writing a book about physicians. Linda was elated because of her years of health care experience and many relationships with physicians. Jim questioned his involvement because his physician contacts were generally limited to annual physicals and occasional infections. How could one write about the medical profession with such limited knowledge?

When we began writing our first book, *Reclaiming Soul In Health Care, Practical Strategies for Revitalizing Providers of Care,*[1] Linda mentioned the project to her personal physician who then proceeded to share his story. Resulting from this interview came an understanding of his journey and himself that never would have occurred without it.

Shortly after Linda concluded the first few tape-recorded interviews, it became perfectly clear that this book was simply going to be a series of captivating stories essentially told by physicians themselves. Our task involved capturing them and including our personal reflections and insights as appropriate. The book's audience would be other physicians who, by reading the book, might connect more deeply to their own passion, resilience, and hope for their profession. If you are a layperson, we believe you will be able to connect with your own physician at a different, more soulful level. The themes are relevant to physicians and indirectly to each of us involved in health care in one manner or another. To illustrate just a few, Bob Barnes' "Uncle Joe," Nancy Neubauer's visiting "angel," and Rhonda Ringer's dance with an Alzheimer patient will enthrall you.

The 33 physician stories in this book evolved, not through a random selection process, but through Linda's contacts, referrals from others, and simply through a physician's own expressions of interest. We interviewed a diverse group in terms of age, gender,

---

[1] Henry LG, Henry JD. *Reclaiming Soul In Health Care, Practical Strategies for Revitalizing Providers of Care.* Chicago, IL: Health Forum, Inc, AHA Press; 1999.

cultural orientation, practice specialty, length of time in practice, and geographic location. When we distributed the questions as included in the section, "Strategies for Caring for Oneself," we soon found that participants already had a bent to them.

We wish our readers could have been present during the interviews. Like e-mail, the written word loses some of the vitality of an intimate face-to-face meeting. It may cause us to oversimplify or generalize too quickly and lock us into fixed, rather than fluid, images. We encourage the reader to continually remind himself or herself that each person's story is open ended and ever evolving. Also, each one of us travels on a dimly lit path in terms of consciousness. The great value of listening to another person's story is that it may enlighten our own journey.

Based on general emphasis, we arranged the stories into eight sections. By doing so, we do not mean to imply that some of the physicians interviewed are not innovators, teachers, cultivators, and the like. These physicians are multiskilled and easily could have been placed in more than one section. We simply wanted to provide some structure to the book.

We express deep appreciation to the people who shared part of their journey with us and to the AMA for bringing them to the public. Special thanks go to Suzanne Fraker, Director, Product Line Development, AMA Press, for her dedication to and enthusiastic support of this project.

INTRODUCTION

At a 1991 conference on the convergence of science and religion, Ruth Barnhouse, MD, offered an imaginative simile about how we humans approach and attempt to understand ultimate truth. Before her retirement and subsequent death in 1999, Dr Barnhouse, an ordained Episcopal priest, served as professor of psychiatry and pastoral care, Perkins School of Theology, Southern Methodist University. She previously had been a clinical assistant in psychiatry at Harvard University and was a Life Fellow of the American Psychiatric Society.

"In seeking absolute truth we aim at the unattainable, and must be content with finding broken portions."

-Sir William Osler, MD
Aequanimitas (1932)

"Imagine that there is a mobile containing a thousand pieces of stained glass, including every conceivable color, size, and shape. The mobile hangs in a doorway. You could sit anywhere indoors or outdoors and look at the mobile for your entire lifetime. With the changing play of the light shining upon it from the sun, moon, and stars and the wind weaving its way through and around the stained glass, it would never look twice the same. And, you could never say you have seen all of it, every single thing about it that was possible to see. Not only this, but at the end of your life, when you had finished sitting there submitting to this experience, you would have to recognize that if you had been sitting only three feet away, you would have had an entirely different experience of the mobile."[1]

Dr Barnhouse then made the point that most theological (and, we might add, many scientific) arguments often strike one as people who are rushing in to take a quick Polaroid picture of the mobile and then running out into another room to fight with each other about whose picture is right. This is simply disrespectful of the universe's complexity.

In his book, *The Way of the Physician*, philosopher, historian, and prolific writer Jacob Needleman brings to light the fact that there are two serpents rather than one in most images of the caduceus,

---

[1] Isthmus Institute, Dallas, Texas. Annual Conference [unpublished videotape]. 1991.

which is widely accepted as the emblem of medicine. He suggests that the two serpents "represent two fundamental forces of universal nature—one moving outward, away from the Source and the second moving back toward union with the Source."[2] However, he suggests that the view of nature held by many scientists is one-dimensional. Nature is seen primarily as secular and mechanical. The second serpent is needed to reintroduce us to the sacred aspect of nature. "The meaning of the art of medicine, like the very meaning of life itself, cannot be found through one force alone."[3] Both forces influence physicians who are deeply connected to soul. This book is about their stories.

Physician, Tell Thy Story

"Everybody is a story. When I was a child, people sat around kitchen tables and told their stories. We don't do that so much anymore. Sitting around the table telling stories is not just a way of passing time. It is the way the wisdom gets passed along."

Rachel Naomi Remen, MD
Kitchen Table Wisdom (1996)

We are told that some physicians see themselves as being terribly isolated. They work long hours. Some are under great pressure to be competitive and to produce. They hesitate to reveal very much about themselves, and especially their emotions, sometimes because of organizational politics. In part, the reluctance may be due to the very hierarchal position of the physician in the care-giving equation. In his book, *Healing the Wounds, A Physician Looks at His Work*, David Hilfiker, MD, reflects on this hierarchy.

"My position as physician automatically conferred upon me an authority that was independent of my abilities. . . . The prestige and authority that accompanied my position as physician seemed initially very attractive, almost adequate rewards in themselves for all the other pressures of the job. In the end, however, they helped to isolate me from the healing relationships with my patients that might have allowed me to handle the stresses of the job in a more balanced way over a longer period of time."[4]

---

[2] Needleman J. *The Way of the Physician,* San Francisco, CA: Harper & Row; 1985: xi.

[3] Needleman J. *The Way of the Physician,* San Francisco, CA: Harper & Row; 1985: xii.

[4] Hilfiker D. *Healing the Wounds, A Physician Looks at His Work.* New York, NY: Penguin Books, Viking Penguin, Inc; 1987: 152–155.

Peter Ways, MD, whom we will introduce later in this book, speaks about having no one available to help him deal with the experience of his first cadaver or the loss of his first patient. Yet, to be human is to have a story. Sharing one's story in a nonjudgmental setting can be enormously healing. As Dr Hilfiker also notes that,

"For his part, the physician often finds it difficult to step down from his usual place of authority and ask for help. . . . The end result is isolation from potentially healing human contact. The physician is left alone with the overwhelming burden of being helper, healer, doer, of conforming to the expectations of 'good men' in our dominant Western Culture. He is ideally always in charge, not swayed by emotion (yet compassionate), efficient, powerful, omniscient. The possibility of sharing is lost, and the physician goes his own way."[5]

This is why a rigorous, time-consuming review of one's life story in the presence of a kind and attentive audience remains central to recovery in 12-step programs. Although not necessarily 12 steps, Caduceus Clubs provide a meeting place where true physician group relationships and therapy are provided. In fact, more and more impaired physicians are joining them as part of their own recovery program.

Although most caregivers are probably wounded healers in one way or another, one does not have to be impaired to benefit from such a group experience. About 6 years ago, Jim participated in a support group of five men that included a neurologist who is heavily involved in treating depression and other disorders through electroencephalograph biofeedback. Working primarily with our dreams, one of us would share a dream and the others would respond by suggesting what it might mean to them if it had been their dream. This provided the dreamer with a wider range of suggestions, expanding personal insight as well as increasing a deep sense of community within the group. Working with dreams acts as a superb means to explore the mysteries of psyche or soul and to recapture one's story.

The importance of storytelling can be seen in many arenas. In his book, *The Healing Art of Storytelling*, Richard Stone takes the reader on an inward journey to relearn the healing art of storytelling. It includes step-by-step explanations of how we can use stories to uncover lost pieces of ourselves, discover places that are

[5] Hilfiker D. *Healing the Wounds, A Physician Looks at His Work*. New York, NY: Penguin Books, Viking Penguin, Inc; 1987: 66.

hidden wellsprings of healing, and satisfy the hunger for meaning in our lives.

> "Through storytelling we can come to know who we are in new and unforeseen ways. We can also reveal to others what is deepest in our hearts and, in the process, build bridges. The very act of sharing a story with another human being contradicts the extreme isolation that characterizes so many of our lives."[6]

Richard used storytelling with a major regional health care system to improve the level of caring for each other and for patients. Taking the time to share and to listen to one another profoundly impacts healthy, respectful, and productive work relationships. It increases empathy with patients' problems, builds a sense of community, and deepens appreciation for diversity among people.

Soliciting stories need not be difficult or time consuming. Jim likes to ask what he calls a 1-minute, soul-connecting question, namely, "What interests you these days?" For example, he asked this question of a physician's assistant during a routine physical exam. Fred (not his real name) promptly explained that he would soon vacation in Hawaii where he had been stationed during his military service as a medic. Then the question was turned back, Fred asking Jim, "What interests *you* these days?" Jim spoke of a recent career discussion with a nurse who was deeply interested in aromatherapy. Whereupon Fred began speaking about how he enjoyed the unique and therapeutic smell of cucumbers. This dialogue, which Jim will always remember, took place within a few, short minutes.

Responses to this simple question demonstrate that most people enjoy telling their stories. In his video recording on the subject of storytelling, Thomas Moore states, "People are hungry for a life which has deep value in it. We can uncover this deep value through storytelling. Stories give us a sense of history."[7] To tell our stories and to have them listened to enrich the soul of an individual and an organization.

Evelyn Clark's consulting business, Corporate Storytelling, is all about capturing authentic business stories and "walking the talk" in terms of marketing them. Successful marketing hinges on

---

[6] Stone R. *The Healing Art of Storytelling.* New York, NY: Hyperion; 1996: 3.

[7] Moore T. *Discovering Everyday Spirituality: Story.* PBS Home Video; 1996.

telling who you are at your core, what you have to offer, and reaching the right people. She created a process for helping organizations get to their core story and discover their values. It becomes a matter of identifying who they are in reality, how they operate, and what drives their decisions. She says,

"It is a matter of helping an organization recall what it was in the past, what it is now, and what it wants to become. Where did it start and how has it changed? Is there a gap between what management believes and what the rank and file employees believe? Then we take a look at what is wanted in terms of the future and communicate that vision internally and externally."

Generally, the process operates the same way for individuals with whom Jim works as part of career assessment. He asks his clients to reflect on key accomplishments throughout their lives from early ages up to the present time. They share stories about what they achieved, specifically about how they achieved, and how they felt about their achievements. From these stories, Jim extracts reoccurring patterns of skills that people are almost compelled to use. Having worked with more than 50 clients over the years, he almost always uncovers a pattern of vocational passion.

In his book, *The Soul's Code*, James Hillman affirms the validity of this approach. He suggests that, just as an acorn knows instinctively what it means to become an oak tree, so too, we have a unique, genetic instinct of what we were placed here on earth to accomplish.

"There is more in a human life than our theories of it allow. Sooner or later something seems to call us onto a particular path. You may remember this 'something' as a signal moment in childhood when an urge out of nowhere, a fascination, a peculiar turn of events struck like an annunciation: This is what I must do, this is what I've got to have. This is who I am."[8]

Connecting Through Stories

Medicine creates a unique relationship between the healer (physician) and the patient. There is almost no other arena where this kind of partnership is found. Many physicians agree on the importance of knowing the whole stories of their patients. Dr David Hilfiker suggests that,

"The blessing and the curse of medicine is that we physicians are privileged to share the most intense moments of life with our patients: birth, death, fear, sorrow, anxiety, disability, healing, joy. These moments are

---

[8] Hillman J. *The Soul's Code*. New York, NY: Random House; 1996: 3.

shared without the usual social barriers; thus we are privy to the deepest of humanity's experiences. But with the privilege comes the burden of availability, of openness to the needs revealed at those intense times."[9]

In fact, good clinical outcomes are enhanced by this holistic approach. We believe that the reverse is also true. The importance of patients knowing the physician's story is equally vital. Sharing stories creates a sense of partnership.

Paradigm Shift
Consider the following story:

> The director of the Denver Zoo was overjoyed with the news. For some time, she had yearned for a polar bear to add to the zoo's population. Now, one had become available and would be delivered within the month. However, there was no suitable place to house the bear, so plans were drawn up immediately to construct a suitable habitat. In the meantime, the polar bear arrived and was placed in a temporary cage.
>
> The cage was only 9-ft wide and 20-ft long. So, day in and day out, the bear paced back and forth within this tiny space. This continued for more than a month, until finally the great day arrived. Both the bear and the cage were moved to his new home, beautifully landscaped with rocks, foliage, and a pond. Then the door of the cage was opened. The bear tentatively walked out, and the cage was removed. He looked around at the strange new surroundings for a short period of time, then began to pace back and forth again within the imaginary confines of a 9-ft by 20-ft space.

The polar bear was a victim of his assumptions. Because he had lived within the limitations of his cage for a great length of time, he assumed the boundaries were still present. Even though the cage was removed and his new home was much more spacious, the bear chose to remain limited by his old confines.

Of course, boundaries are important and vital to our well-being. Without any boundaries (eg, walls, road and traffic signs and systems), we would experience chaos. However, invisible boundaries, assumptions, and belief systems also influence us. Like the bear in the cage, we assume certain things, even though these assumptions may no longer be appropriate or functional. For example, as a career consultant, Jim has worked with many people helping them to assess their career interests and strengths.

---

[9] Hilfiker D. *Healing the Wounds: A Physician Looks at His Work.* New York, NY: Penguin Books, Viking Penguin, Inc; 1987: 37.

Then he encourages people to take control of their careers and work situations because with the increasing number of mergers, acquisitions, reengineering, downsizing, and layoffs, job security is a thing of the past. Yet, many people remain frozen in denial, assuming that change won't affect them. It is the bear-in-the-cage syndrome, living and moving within a boundary system that no longer functions or exists.

"We must always change, review and rejuvenate ourselves, or we harden."

-Johann Goethe

Today our society remains bound within invisible barriers established originally by the perceptions of philosophers and scientists some 300 years ago. Throughout human history, up until the seventeenth century, cultures all over the earth existed in what we might call an "enchanted world," a world largely based on a different set of beliefs than exist today. People believed that the natural world was filled with mystery, a living community infused with the presence of spirit. Rocks, trees, rivers, and clouds were all seen as wondrous, interconnected, and alive. The vast majority of people viewed nature as a sacred reality that needed to be respected and sometimes offered it gifts and sacrifices to ensure cosmic harmony.

With the dawn of what might be called the "Modern" or "Scientific" Age in Europe, a new perception of the universe began to replace the "enchanted" one in Western civilization. The work of three men—Francis Bacon, René Descartes, and Sir Isaac Newton—especially helped shape the modern "scientific method." With this new perception, the world was viewed not as filled with mystery, but as an objective, quantifiable place. They said that matter and motion interact according to universal, mechanical laws, whose operations can be observed and predicted with mathematical precision.

Sir Isaac Newton, who discovered gravity, came up with the famous concept that the world is a huge clock. God is like the Master Clockmaker, who created the whole complex mechanism and set all of its work in motion. Then God withdrew and let it run on its own.

This belief (paradigm) continues to dominate our thinking patterns and actions today. Everything is to be conquered, used, or manipulated. It results in a disenchantment and disconnection from the earth. It often results in becoming alienated from each other and from true community.

The Universe as a Living, Energized Tapestry of Relationships[10]

However, today, just as we have turned the century, the worldview is changing again. The brief period that historians call the "Modern Age" is coming to an end. Many scientists, and especially those in the field of theoretical physics, tell us that the universe can no longer be viewed as a system of independent and inanimate parts. Rather, because of the indivisibility of quantum action, the universe is better understood as a living, undivided whole. It is more like a symphony. It is a tapestry of relationships. Each string of the tapestry is connected to the whole.

This viewpoint thoroughly nullifies a common belief in American culture that we can all go around "doing our own thing" without regard for our impact on others. It also challenges the belief that what we do in our private lives is of no business to others. Both spiritual and quantum perceptions of the universe suggest that, to some degree, mysteriously, *everything* we do impacts everyone and everything else. The Golden Rule takes on enormous significance in this respect.

Rhythmic Web and Soul

In its December 31, 1999, issue, *Time* magazine selected Albert Einstein as the person of the twentieth century and featured an article on theoretical physics. The article described matter as composed of atoms, which are made of protons, neutrons, and electrons. Electrons can't be divided further, but protons and neutrons are both made of three tinier particles called "quarks." It appears that quarks are multidimensional entities called "branes," some of which manifest themselves as tiny loops of "string."

In our book, *Reclaiming Soul in Health Care*, we introduce the "web" as a simile for soul. We speak, not of an electronic image such as the World Wide Web, but of a mysterious, living, organic phenomenon serving as a unifying energy throughout the universe. And, the strings of the web vibrate!

In 1991, Jim attended a conference on the convergence of religion and science. One of the speakers was Dr John Hagelin, a brilliant, Harvard-trained theoretical physicist. Dr Hagelin went

---

[10] We are indebted to Dr Kathlyn James, Senior Pastor of the First United Methodist Church, Seattle, Washington, for some of this imagery.

to the blackboard and for 20 minutes sketched out a series of mathematical equations related to quantum mechanics, few of which any of the participants could grasp. Finally, he turned to the audience, pointed at the formulations, and said, "Now, what this means is that God is music."

Later in the conference, another speaker stated that Dr Hagelin's remarks reminded her of Sergey Rachmaninoff. Someone asked Sergey how he came to write his music. He said, "It's quite simple. I go into a room, sit down by myself, and listen to the music. When it stops, I write it down."

Music elicits a universal response in people and serves as a collective means of communication. Music engages most of our senses and certainly a wide range of emotion. So, the underlying dynamic of the universe might just be an interconnected tapestry of rhythmic energy. Robert Cole, MD, reports on a study performed at the University of Valencia on the positive impact of music.

> "One hundred and one babies [were provided] with taped violin sounds, arranged from simple to more complex forms, for up to 90 minutes per day beginning at about 28 weeks of gestation. Mothers exposed their babies to the music for an average total of 70 hours. At 6 months of age, the babies in the experimental group were significantly advanced in their motor skills, linguistic development, sensory coordination, and cognitive development when compared with controls."[11]

In many ways, connecting through storytelling is a form of music. We weave our stories, one with another, much as a dance is choreographed to music. Each person takes a part and contributes to a magnificent chorus.

In the following pages we share the stories of physicians whom we interviewed that capture where they are at this moment in time. We find many of the same threads of thought and beliefs expressed among their stories, regardless of their experience or specialty. Their stories reflect three major themes: passion, resilience, and hope.

Included in the section Strategies for Caring for Oneself is a sample of the kinds of questions we asked physicians. Whenever appropriate, we added material to expand on their insights and to provide practical strategies that might be helpful to physicians and laypeople alike.

---

[11] Cole RL. *The Gentle Greeting*. Naperville, IL: Sourcebooks; 1998: 101.

To the best of our ability, during our interviews, we attempted to capture some of the same passion Jim finds in helping people identify their vocational passion. The importance of this enthusiasm and vocational passion is critical to the resiliency of physicians. As Gregg Levoy states in his book, *Callings, Finding and Following an Authentic Life*, "Passion is a state of love, and hunger. It is also a state of enthusiasm . . . we move toward a kind of divine presence because, through our passion, we are utterly present."[12]

We also wanted to uncover ways in which physicians show resilience in the midst of today's accelerating change in health care. Hope especially makes it possible to be resilient. Ultimately, this is a book of hope—the most potent and positive faculty of the physician. The physician (and patient) hopes the diagnosis is correct and the treatment will work. Having hope allows us to forge ahead in spite of current uncertainty and chaos. This book engages a similar hope for the future of the healing professions.

---

[12] Levoy G. *Callings, Finding and Following an Authentic Life*. New York, NY: Harmony Books; 1997: 10.

CULTIVATORS

"He is the best physician who is the most ingenious inspirer of hope."
— Samuel Taylor Coleridge

Medicine as Sacred Journey

Don Greggain, MD, CCFP

A trip is not a journey. When beginning a trip, we generally know where we are going and why. We can estimate the amount of time required to arrive at our destination and decide when to return. But a journey is different. A journey is a quest. It involves seeking answers to questions; it is the "quest-I'm-on." Why am I here? Where am I going? To what end is this quest? As such, by its essential nature, a journey engages us in mystery, wonder, and paradox.

"When you're on a journey, and the end keeps getting further and further away, then you realize that the real end is the journey."

— Karlfried Graf Durckheim
The Path of Initiation (1991)

In many ways, health care is both a trip and a journey. When afflicted with a sinus infection, we make a trip to the physician to receive treatment and hopefully to be cured. Health care is also a journey in the sense that overcoming disease never ceases to end. Whether physical, emotional, or spiritual, we never achieve health in the broadest sense of the word. In one sense, it is like a spiral. Each ending initiates a new beginning, but at a different level. We cure one disease while at the same moment we begin or continue work on another.

For family medicine physician Dr Don Greggain, medical practice can be characterized as a journey. "Life is a journey that we [myself and my patients] are all sharing together. You can't cheat and read the last page first. Each page of life represents a great opportunity."

When asked what the word *soul* means to him, he expressed it this way: " I think soul is a gift from God, an opportunity to enjoin oneself with a higher being. It connects you to something more expansive, to something beyond oneself." His remarks reflect the ancient belief that the soul is not in the body, but the body is in the soul.

Listening to Don's obvious enthusiasm about his practice, we suspected that he experiences much mystery and wonder in his family practice. He affirmed this by commenting, "I experience it every single day! In particular, the beginnings and endings of life always fill me with wonder and mystery—conception, birth, and

3

the magic of bringing new life into the earth. I think of how many things could go wrong; birth is said to be the everyday miracle, and I really believe that."

With obvious emotion, Don talks about death. "Wonder and mystery also embrace the end of life. I see the wisdom, peace, and serenity of my older patients. I sit at my patients' bedsides and experience them dying, and often it is uncanny. I have a woman dying this week. She was active and vibrant until recently, and then hastily went downhill. Her husband became ill also, probably from exhaustion. I think she should have died a couple of nights ago. But, I think she chose not to die until she was confident that he would be all right. Great wisdom often surfaces during these times, and I am greatly honored to be part of the experience."

Don's journey into medicine began with the encouragement of his sixth-grade schoolteacher. Long before selecting this career, his teacher must have sensed his love for the sciences and his delight in being among a group of people.

"Listen for things that speak themselves."

— Patricia Monaghan
Winter-Burning (1991)

"I don't remember the conversation in particular, other than her saying that medicine would be a perfect match for me. She planted a seed that germinated over a period of time. I think that I had an aptitude for medicine and by the time I actually applied to medical school, I did believe that I was born to be in medicine."

However, his mother was horrified by the notion that he might enter this profession and actually cried when he announced his intentions. With the birth and subsequent death of her first child, Don's mother had a very bad experience with a physician who colored her perception of the medical field. "I don't for a moment believe that this doctor was responsible for the tragedy, but she still has not really forgiven that man. So it took her a little while to accept the notion of my entering medicine."

Like most physicians, Don possesses an intense desire to do well in his chosen profession. He believes that a good physician essentially educates and communicates with compassion.

"Compassion involves sharing from the heart, being empathetic, and having a desire to understand," he says. Apart from his technical knowledge and skill, effective medicine for him involves viewing the patient–physician relationship as one of exchanging information.

"My patients share information about what is occurring in their lives and how they feel about it. In turn, I interpret it and provide feedback. I give them the tools to make choices. But it's not simply providing information about medical procedures and interventions. In a broader sense, it involves the sharing of two lives."

He realizes that there are limitations, some of which are time imposed and others determined by how much a person is willing to share. Also, he understands that everyone has different perceptions and ways of interpreting life events. "Of course, in long-term relationships we learn more of another person's story," he says. "I had a long-term relationship with my grandmother. However, when I attended her funeral, I had no idea of some of her gifts and talents that were eulogized by others."

He shares parts of his own life story on a regular basis with patients, depending on their situation. "I find it extremely helpful to share my story. It could be the sharing of an experience similar to that which the patient is facing. I may have had a family illness comparable to his or hers. In other instances, the story may have nothing to do with medicine, but simply reflect who and what I am as a person. In reality, even the art hanging on the wall or the type of people we physicians hire communicates to some degree who we are as persons."

Don attributes much of who he is to his father. "My father was and still is my hero. My father worked as a tire salesman, so he was gone much of the time. My mother was probably the most important parental influence in my life in terms of developing values and a work ethic. She was responsible for my success in terms of the skills developed during adolescence."

"However, my father always had an incredible capacity to make people feel special. He made us feel that we are a part of something bigger and better than any one person. He has no capacity to be selfish. He would drive hundreds of miles to be home for a basketball game in which I played, even though I wasn't a star player. I just knew that when I was on the court and I looked up in the stands, that my father would be there."

During his father's working life, it was nothing for his father to get up during the night and go out to help someone who had a tire problem. In fact, even after he retired, a truck driver called in the middle of the night asking him to change a tire.

"Also, he always taught me how to love my wife by my seeing how he loves his wife. I grew up thinking that all men washed dishes, cooked meals, and did housework. When I dated and married my wife, she said that my father was the first person of his generation who she ever saw do such things. So my father is my hero."

Don attended medical school in Canada. Because other physicians interviewed for this book mentioned it, we asked Don whether he found the experience of formal medical training abusive in one form or another. He said, "I believe that abuse is a role that one chooses to accept or not to accept. We worked many, ungodly hours, but I would say that my family suffered much more than I did. I was married and had children while attending medical school. Often absent from home, I was saddened to miss much of the early years of my children. But I took delight in my education. I attended a teaching hospital limited to family medicine residents. I loved the opportunity to learn. I suppose in a philosophical way, working 24-hour shifts was abusive, but at the time I didn't feel mistreated. I was too excited to be in that environment."

During the interview, Don spoke with delight about his son, who at the time was just entering medical school to become a pediatrician. "Joshua has been a 'kid magnet' for all of his life. We don't know why, but children love him. For almost 6 months during a period of unrest, he visited Africa on the Ivory Coast and on the border of Liberia. Because he could speak both English and French, he worked with Liberian refugees fleeing from that country. Joshua would enter the villages to help improve safe water resources and to provide some education. Because they had never seen a white person before and thought he was a kind of bogeyman, the children would all disappear when he came to a village. Once he was able to overcome their fear, the children began to flock to him. God has blessed him with the particular gifts of relating to children."

Don believes that he has changed as a physician over the years. "I'm less of a know-it-all. I don't need to be right all of the time. I don't need to be resentful about other people's choices or mistakes, nor do I need to feel responsible for my patients' decisions. I am an educator and communicator, but I'm not their mother. Earlier, I may have had an artificial notion of self-importance, which we often bring with us from medical school. Today, I am more respectful of my patients."

For example, Don speaks of a middle-aged man who had recently attempted suicide. He said that 20 years ago he would have been very angry with him, asking why such a person would want to waste so much potential. "Instead, I [today] was simply saddened. And, so was he. He was saddened by what he had done the previous night. I was worried about sending him home, where he might attempt suicide again. But, in the end, he must take responsibility for his actions."

Over time, physicians make mistakes. In her book, *Unity of Mistakes*, Tracy Paget states, "Medical mistakes are an intrinsic feature of medical work."[1] We asked Don how he handles clinical errors. He said, "In the same way that most people handle it when they make mistakes. It's a grief process. It's been said that a foolish man does not learn from his mistakes. On the other hand, an intelligent man learns from his mistakes and a wise man learns from other people's mistakes. One of the most poignant lessons I've learned during the practice of medicine is to learn from my mistakes and not to repeat them. Also, I've learned that these days if you have not made a commitment to lifelong learning, you cannot be an effective physician."

The importance of being resilient in the midst of change was born out by Don's life. A second generation Canadian, one of Don's most difficult life decisions resulted in his leaving his birth country. Believing that the health care system in Alberta was ill, in 1995 he moved from Canada to a small rural US community. He is convinced that the Canadian system failed its constituents. Even though he had many dear friends in Alberta and two teenagers in high school, he decided to walk away from this medical climate.

"During the late 80s and early 90s I worked very actively with the Alberta Medical Association, trying to find new ways of providing health care, making it more cost effective and affordable. The political powers encouraged us to pursue these avenues. When we came close to what we believed was a reasonable long-term resolution, we were told that our solutions didn't conform to their political agenda. Thereafter, health care budgets were reduced by 40% and we were told to send hospitalized patients back to their homes. It was a tragedy and I had dying people placed on waiting lists, waiting to see a cardiologist or to enter oncology treatment."

---

[1] Paget T. *Unity of Mistakes*. Philadelphia, PA: Temple University Press; 1988: 15.

He recalls his increasingly intense feelings of frustration. "One day my daughter asked why I didn't laugh much anymore. She was right, and this was not how I wanted to spend my life. I knew that something had to change. I had to give up the sacred cow of my birthplace and move to America."

Don believes, for all of its faults, the US health care system remains excellent. "Like every system, it needs some work. It may need to be more compassionate and to spend more tax dollars to help the millions of people who are not privileged with coverage, but it is the best in the world."

Contrary to some others in the profession, Don remains very optimistic about health care. "I am perhaps pathologically optimistic," he says. "I see in the medical profession such creativity, ingenuity, and intelligence. The opportunity to do good gets better with each passing year."

"I am also encouraged when I hear people speak about the need to address poverty. I hear people saying that poverty is dictated by health. I believe it is just the opposite; health is dictated by poverty. The more impoverished you are, the less likely you are to be healthy. There is a direct correlation with rising standards of living in the world and longevity. To be able to contribute to this possibility of doing good in this day and age is a privilege."

Don says that it saddens him to hear of physicians who throw up their hands in today's changing environment and talk about leaving the profession. "Such negativity is one perspective; another is to be creative and find new ways of providing care. Medicine, like other professions, embraces a diverse population," he reminds us. "Some people are optimists and some pessimists. Some are very creative, while others are rather traditional. Medicine embraces them all. So if we are not waking up in the morning delighted by the opportunity to care for patients, then we should find something else to do or move to a different environment."

Don reflects on the end of his journey and what he would like others to say about his life at its end. "I hope my patients would say that I was a man of God who cared for them in a personal way. I would like them to say that I shared my heart with them, that what I have pursued was not simply a job. My goal in life is that no matter whom I encounter, it is not simply about me but about something that is much broader."

He concludes by saying, "In terms of medicine, someone once said that medicine is the art of entertaining the patient while God does the healing. It is a little tongue-in-cheek to suggest that doctors should entertain patients, but we do try to give them opportunities to use things that might make them better. But God does the healing."

Gentle Greeter

John Gollhofer, MD

In his book, *The Gentle Greeting*, Ronald Cole, MD, coaches his support team to

> "never underestimate the importance of letting the laboring mother know that she is loved and supported. I will never forget the comment one of the support team members made [after a contraction]. . . . The expectant woman said, 'That was a tough one.' Her team member whispered to her, 'That means he is getting closer and closer to your arms.'"[2]

We perceive obstetrician Dr John Gollhofer to be such a gentle greeter.

John is a member of a 140-physician multispecialty group with clinics in and around the Spokane, Washington, area. His office is in one of the main clinic locations and sits atop a seven-story garage/medical office building with a panoramic view of the city. A practicing physician for some 22 years, he remembers backing into medicine. Grinning, he says, "I wasn't smart enough to be a nuclear physicist, so I decided to become a physician. It was a very lucky or perhaps it was a divine accident that it worked out this way. I say this because I really love what I do. I was good in science and enjoyed the various disciplines. However, I wasn't quite smart enough to be a physicist. I just couldn't understand matrix algebra. The professor confirmed this and said that I *never* would understand it. He said he would give me a 'B' in the class if I promised never to take another math course," he laughs. "That left me with molecular biology, and I excelled in it."

Specializing in obstetrics and gynecology seemed to be a good match. "I enjoy dealing with largely healthy people as opposed to those who have chronic or critical illnesses. Also, in medical school I had some professors who impressed me with their character. There is a certain amount of hero patterning involved with doctors whom one respects," he adds. "In addition, I enjoy delivering babies more than any other aspect of my practice. It's not difficult to do if you are having fun."

Having fun delivering babies is only part of the enjoyment John finds in his practice. His conversation is generously

---

[2] Cole RL. *The Gentle Greeting*. Naperville, IL: Sourcebooks; 1998: 101.

peppered with patient stories that reflect the wonder and mystery he often experiences. He recalls one such story.

"I had a patient who phoned us because she was experiencing decreased fetal movement. We get calls like this all the time, and we evaluate them. Most often, there is nothing wrong with the fetus, but we always respond. At 26 weeks of pregnancy, you are not supposed to have consistent movement. It was a Saturday, and I asked her to come to the hospital for an evaluation. At the time, I thought it was another false alarm. However, on examination, the heart tones were not quite normal, so we performed an ultrasound that, indeed, turned out to be abnormal. The baby was not moving."

"The perinatologist on call that day and I put our heads together, discussing the fact that what was occurring didn't make any sense. We ordered another test to determine whether there were fetal blood cells in the maternal circulation. The test was positive, implying that there had been a transfusion from the fetus to the mother, which theoretically can happen. It suggested that the fetus was profoundly anemic, causing the problem. So we returned to the ultrasound, and my associate scanned it for about an hour because neither of us could hardly believe what was occurring."

John remembers them agonizing over the decision. "We didn't know what to do next, because delivering a baby after only 26 weeks is considerably premature. If we were wrong in our diagnosis, the baby might not survive. Still, we did a C-section and delivered the baby, who turned out to be profoundly anemic. I had no idea how this child survived. However, the perinatologist pulled the baby through the crisis."

He adds happily, "I just got word that the child is doing quite well at 10 months of age and is normal. It was one of those diagnostic dilemmas where we did all of the things we probably should have done without necessarily having any definitive reason to do them. If during any step along the way we had lost faith with the process, saying that it didn't make sense to perform a 26-week cesarean section, it would have had a fatal outcome. The fact that the baby turned out to be well is almost too happy an ending for the story. One senses that it may have been divine guidance that made the process turn out the way it did. In any case, we witnessed a mystery because there was no scientific process leading us to take such an action. We acted like doctors based upon our best knowledge, but something else was involved."

John is reminded of a second story. During a difficult delivery, the baby had his shoulders stuck in the mother's pelvis. Such a complication often leads to fetal injury and even death. "There are a number of maneuvers that one can perform to deliver the shoulder," he says. "Basically, I tried all of them, but none of them worked. At that point, there was only one maneuver I hadn't attempted, bringing the arm out in a manner that is anatomically impossible and really shouldn't work. But, I said a little prayer, did the maneuvering, and out popped the arm. When something happens that scientifically isn't supposed to happen, I think that is a miracle. There is no other way to explain it."

"A person's a person, no matter how small."

— Dr Seuss
Oh, The Places You'll Go (1990)

As with most physicians, John has had major setbacks and readily admits to dealing with his own grief. "I had a baby with an avulsed cord during delivery. It was a freak occurrence where all of the blood vessels were on the membranes. A baby's head will typically slip past those blood vessels. In this case, it was somewhat like a net. The baby exsanguinated before it was born, and we could not resuscitate the child. Frankly, the patient herself got me through the grief. She understood that everything was done that could have been done. She was very grateful and very supportive of our efforts."

Many, if not most, physicians admit that processing their personal grief can be especially difficult because of their role as physician. Even while feeling loss, there is an expectation of immediately moving on, relating to the next patient who expects 100% of his or her attention. John agrees. "It is very difficult, but at the same time, that's what defines a professional caregiver. We need to function in some manner regardless of the condition of our emotions. Of course, there are some days better than others, but we must be able to function at a level commensurate with one's level of competence."

David Hilfiker, MD, talks about the wrenching reality of moving from one patient to another even in the midst of personal pain. After pronouncing a child dead, he writes, "I feel a churning inside. On a better day, I know I could empathize with Mrs Williams's (chronic complainer) pain, with her emptiness. . . . And, she would leave feeling a little better simply because I'd paid attention. But today isn't a better day. I'm tired, grieving over Ricky's death, concerned for Joan [mother]. I can't find the energy."[3]

John is particularly sensitive to helping his patients to process grief. When a pregnant woman suffers a miscarriage, he counsels with her about dealing with her grief and loss. Hearing the importance he places on acknowledging and dealing with grief, we are reminded of the book, *Welcoming the Soul of a Child*, by Jill E. Hopkins, MA. Among the various rituals she describes are those that are appropriate when experiencing any loss, including that of a fetus or newborn baby. One such ritual is the ancient practice of planting a tree honoring a rite of passage.

She suggests opening the ritual by stating its purpose. It might go something like this: "Today, I come to this place on my healing path, where I willingly and lovingly honor, release, and free myself of this particular pain and loss." She then suggests taking a symbol of the loss, putting it in a ceremonial space, and imagining that it contains the grief, hurt, or anger to be released. When ready, blow three breaths into the symbol, and then place it in a piece of cloth or paper bag. It then can be discarded in the trash or burned later. She then advises saying something that prepares the way for healing and new life, similar to: "In letting go of the grief, I now make a healthy, nourishing, and loving environment in my body and in my life for my future child. I invite this child into my (our) life now." Then, plant a tree while thinking of the soil, the oxygen, the sun, and the water as nutrients for that which is wished to grow. Finally, she suggests expressing gratitude to all the elements, to oneself for doing the ritual, followed by giving thanks to whomever and whatever you feel assists you on your healing path.[4]

As a physician today, John believes he has grown over time, especially in terms of his faith. "I have a much stronger faith in God and His workings," he says. "I believe in spirituality and mysticism, but we are not encouraged to speak about such things as practitioners. As outgoing president of the Washington State

---

[3] Hilfiker D. *Healing the Wounds: A Physician Looks at His Work*. New York, NY: Penguin Books, Viking Penguin, Inc; 1987: 24–25.

[4] Hopkins JE. Foreword by Kornfield J. *Welcoming the Soul of a Child, Creating Rituals and Ceremonies to Honor the Birth of Our Sons and Daughters*. New York, NY: Kensington Books, Kensington Publishing Corp; 1999: 69–70.

Medical Association, I will give a farewell address. If I gave a speech based upon the interview questions you are asking me, the majority of the audience would be quite uncomfortable. I don't mean this in a critical sense; there are simply some topics that are very private. Spirituality is one of these subjects. Apart from TV evangelists, most people are private about their faith and spirituality."

Much of what has changed over time directly relates to medical care. "Every day, doctors must let go of procedures and treatments no longer working for them," John asserts. "What we do today is not anything like what we did 20 years ago. This includes what we do during deliveries as well as the treatment of certain diseases. Ectopic pregnancies serve as an excellent example. Technology has totally changed the way we manage this condition. When I began, miscarriages were diagnosed when a pregnancy test went from positive to negative, which usually didn't occur until after tissue was passed. Before a first symptom appears, now miscarriages are diagnosed through the use of ultrasound. So, it is a matter of giving up old strategies and embracing new knowledge and technologies."

John describes a good physician as someone who is patient-centered. "A good doctor cares more about the patient than he or she does about himself or any other aspect of life, whether that be family members, a bank account, prestige, or anything else. Good doctors care more about the patient than any other aspect of the profession. It makes it easy to practice medicine. If you worked for Microsoft or some other nonhealth care group, you might sometimes wonder what the mission of the organization truly is. However, in medicine it is quite simple. It involves taking care of patients."

Active listening is also the mark of a good physician. John acknowledges that today he is a much better listener than when he started. He believes, unfortunately, that this is a skill physicians were not trained to develop during medical school or residency.

"Obviously, you must listen if you are going to be competent in diagnosis and treatment. I've really learned to hear what people are telling me, because often they will tell you things that are not explicit. If you haven't learned the skill of active listening, you will not do as well as you could. Usually patients know what is wrong with them or will tell you what they think is the problem. If you listen, eventually you will get the information that you need. This is why our medical sages have always told us that diagnosis is tied 90% of the time to history taking. Taking a patient's history is an art."

Beyond his technical expertise, John considers his own essential skills to include personally and deeply caring for another person coupled with a desire to ensure that the patient has a good outcome from a medical problem. "I'm a perfectionist. I do things the right way, including completing the paperwork."

With the changes taking place in health care today, we asked John to address his view of the future of health care. "In one sense I am hopeful because we have many good people who are patient-centered and who are attempting to help those who are in need. In addition, technology and funding are available to continue in this manner. I can't believe that our society is going to turn its back on quality health care in the name of cost control. People will always support the healing arts and the people who practice them."

"On the other hand, I believe that we are currently going through a very difficult transition. There is a certain economic hierarchy in this culture. To some extent, there should be; if you have money you get services and goods and that's fine. But, we are going to have to figure out a way to provide services to those without the funds. I think we will eventually do this, but we are in the midst of a swing of the pendulum. For example, on the positive side, organizations like the Gates Foundation are funding immunizations for the poor. This is just the beginning. We may even begin providing services like we had many years ago where people with a need could come without cost."

Some people lament the passing of a period in medicine described as the "golden age of medicine." To this, John replies, "I would describe the golden age of medicine as a period when physicians were supreme authorities and enjoyed a very lucrative, guaranteed income. As this environment disintegrates and physicians lose their incomes and leave their practices, those remaining are focused upon caring for patients. I'm not saying that doctors who are greatly frustrated with today's health care climate don't care about their patients. And, we will lose some of our finest minds if we say to someone that if you enter the medical profession, all you will get out of it is the ability to practice with compassion and make a difference in someone's life."

In the midst of so much change caused by managed care and accelerating regulation, John advises other physicians to keep their eye on the fundamental purpose of medicine. "It involves remembering why we are in the profession. If the circumstances under which we practice medicine are driving someone crazy, well, we need to refocus upon our mission. I understand that the current system doesn't meet anyone's needs, but it is the system that we have. On the other hand, I never take lightly the reality that doctors and patients are suffering because of it. We may reach a time when we simply cannot function any more. It may happen that too much pressure is applied. For example, if I were a primary care physician having to deal with all of the insurance company authorizations and having to answer their queries, I might feel very differently about practicing medicine."

"In OB/GYN, especially with the women's health care access law in the state of Washington, I don't necessarily have a lot of third-party pressure. My life is not nearly as bad as the lives of some others. Some doctors are leaving medicine because they can't afford to keep their doors open anymore. That is a whole different aspect of the practice. If, in spite of your best efforts, your practice is losing money, you have no choice but to close it down. I can see that if you placed your heart and soul in your practice for 25 years and today it is insolvent, you might just quit medicine altogether. There is probably more of this happening than we know of because doctors are not going to advertise the fact that they have just gone into bankruptcy."

"To exist is to change, to change is to mature, to mature is to go on creating oneself endlessly."

— Henri Bergson
Creative Evolution (1911)

"I have a nephew who is about 30 years old. He graduated from college and was an officer in the Marines. Now he works in food service and was managing a fast-food breakfast place. When my brother was on the phone a few years ago, he told me that my nephew got a promotion and is now managing two of these waffle houses and is making $80,000 a year. I told my brother how that was wonderful news. On the other hand, I realize that some doctors practicing primary care in my area would be happy to make $60,000 a year. And, they are working 80 or more hours a week. I think to myself, 'What kind of crazy system do we have in the country where a manager of two waffle restaurants can make more money than a primary care physician? What if the differential were $30,000 or $40,000?

Would doctors start leaving the practice and start managing waffle houses?'"

"At some point you go where your services are valued. If we as a society continue to undervalue the doctor's services, I don't know if we are going to have many of them, or at least many good physicians. You also could say the same thing about school-teachers. Most teach because they love it. But look at the number of them who are no longer in the education system."

Thinking back to his own experience as a medical student, John addresses the examples of abusive medical training reported by some physicians. "You must understand that I am a white male who attended an Ivy League college. I was not a person who was likely to be abused. I knew how to get along with people and had a reasonable northern European external appearance."

"I don't recall seeing others being abused or being humiliated in public. On the other hand, most people never complained about it or would not admit being mistreated. But, I've heard stories from very credible people. It seems like the stories I hear from female practitioners are enough to make your skin crawl."

"Putting it differently, during the past 10 years there have been some minor situations of abuse laid upon me by some physicians in positions of authority. Some people are motivated by power and they will tend to use and abuse it. We need to be careful about putting people in leadership positions who are driven by power as a main reward. However, most physicians are patient-oriented and not power-oriented."

"If you engage in violence [abuse] now, you probably were hit, shaken, yelled at, damaged or broken when you were a baby. Too tiny to defend yourself, you could only absorb it."

— Elaine Childs-Gowell, Good Grief Rituals (1992)

"Where I do sometimes experience abuse is from some patients and from patients' families. Part of the magic of medicine is empowering patients and their families. If you empower people who are essentially good, it serves to bring out the best in them. On the other hand, if you attempt to empower some others, it simply makes them become abusive. For example, when you say that you are sorry about being late for an appointment, most people will accept the apology. However, others can become quite critical of you and/or your office personnel. You simply have to accept this as their way of dealing with the world. Some patients seem to enjoy the role of the bully."

John has no plans to quit practicing medicine any time soon. As he puts it, "As long as my physical and mental skills remain workable, I plan to continue my work as an OB/GYN. I am 54 years old, so I question myself frequently in terms of how well I am performing as a doctor. So far, the answer is positive and I hope this will continue for a long period of time. Money is not a reward in and of itself. Most people who have a passion for their work and who excel at it don't do it for the money. We have to make money along the way in order to support our families and ourselves. But if I weren't able to make enough money to keep my doors open and to send the kids to college, then, of course, I would have to find something else to do. That's a no-brainer. So it's not about money, but we need the money to make the system work."

John has one hero. "My wife is my hero," he says admiringly. "Without complaining, she selflessly and tirelessly makes a wonderful home for my two daughters and me. She is second in line after my patients, but never grumbles about it. It requires a lot of tolerance and patience. What is a hero other than someone who sacrifices him or herself for the greater, external good?"

John concludes by sharing a couple of favorite quotations from two musical rock-and-roll groups. The first is from Nazareth: "History shows again and again how nature points out the folly of man—Godzilla." The second is from The Grateful Dead: "Sometimes the lights all shine on me and other times I can barely see. Lately it's occurred to me what a long, strange trip it's been."

Passion and Sacrifice

Tahmineh Abbasian, MD

To her friends and colleagues, soft-spoken pediatrician Tahmineh Abbasian, MD, is simply Dr Holly. Admitting that her name is difficult to pronounce, the staff say affectionately, "We just call her Dr Holly."

Passion for Holly involves sacrifice. "Passion includes being able to sacrifice everything for which you strive. It embraces the love and motivation to be able to sacrifice for more important things in life," she says gently. Closely related with passion is her perception of soul. "Soul manifests itself through passion and love for life."

Originally from Iran, Holly's path to medicine began at an early age. The medical conditions of two close family members triggered her desire to enter the profession. After attending medical school in Iran, she completed her residency and fellowship at Chicago's Cook County Hospital. As we have remarked in other places in this book, some people believe that medical school can be more difficult for women. Not only was Holly a female going into medicine, but also she had a different cultural background. However, she found her training to be very positive.

Acknowledging the potential challenges, she says, "I think generally being a female in the medical field requires a lot of sacrifice. It makes it harder because many females want to have a family life. Being a mother, managing a household, and at the same time being a professional are quite a challenge."

Holly found herself drawn to pediatrics and neonatology during her medical school pediatrics rotation. "I really enjoyed neonatology for many years, but it became too demanding on my family life," she admits. "So, I decided to limit my practice to pediatrics to have more time to spend with my family." Today, both of her daughters seem interested in the medical field. In fact, on the day of our visit, her older daughter, Javaneh, a college junior, was shadowing her mother.

Holly believes that having a core understanding of spirituality makes a difference in the way she practices medicine and cares for patients. "Since I have a spiritual base from which to operate, it shows in caring for people, being sensitive to their pain and suffering and just being with them as a person more than as a professional." She thinks these are important qualities whatever one's profession. "You can have a healing relationship with a person and not be a doctor. You can just be a friend to a person who is in pain and who is suffering. So, a part of a physician's spirituality is being wholeheartedly present with your patient."

Although not necessarily framed in the language of spirituality, Holly reports that some of her patients have discussed spiritual issues with her. She explains, "I have a patient who, unfortunately, doesn't have much of a chance to become a mother. She only had one pregnancy, and it led to a premature birth. The infant ended up being mentally and physically disabled. But because of her love for her child, I don't think she really sees all of his disabilities. She tells me that Jesus is looking after him and he's going to walk and talk. I allow special time with her because I know she wants me to see the progress he makes, even if it has been limited. It's a special time for the two of us."

Holly's stories are filled with wonder and mystery. She speaks of one in particular that shook her as a physician.

"I had a 22-year-old woman delivering in this hospital 8 or 9 years ago. The mother was young and had no understanding of what I was telling her. Her baby was sick, and I couldn't bring myself to tell her that her baby practically had little chance of surviving. It was the middle of the night when I went to her room, and we could hardly see each other under a very dim light. I told her about the baby's prognosis. She said, 'I know my baby is in your hands and is going to be fine.' I was young myself. She felt that I was a friend and we talked and cried together. I could only tell her, just pray; we both have to pray."

"I sent the baby to another hospital, the only center where they had heart–lung machines. This child was so sick that they had to put him on that machine for over a week. But he survived, even though all of the data suggested that he should have had some brain damage or at least some setback," she says with awe, shaking her head. "He still comes to me; he's in third grade and he is the most intelligent kid in his age group. He had no setback! It's a miracle. Every time I think about it, I get goose bumps. And this is the miracle of life. Since then she has had three other children who are healthy."

Sitting together with the mothers of her patients, woman to woman, is a usual occurrence for Holly. Talking about prayer is also a part of her practice. She says, "Always when I bring bad news to parents, I let them know that not only are we, as physicians, doing the best we can, but that they can get help from whomever is the focus of their faith. "Just pray," she advises. "I think that gives them so much more strength, that they don't have to look to us as the only source of hope. And, it offers them the freedom to talk about their beliefs."

Although such experiences are not infrequent, no one has directly asked her to pray for them. "I don't hear that directly from them, but I know they see that in me. They know that I wish the best for their kids." She is reminded of another story.

"Again, I had another mom who delivered a child with a very primitive heart structure, where the chance of survival for him was practically nonexistent. This child had to go through three different long open-heart surgeries. And, now he is 4½, almost in kindergarten. His mom and I talked in the office, and we prayed for him." Holly believes his mother needed to know that she shared the same feeling about the child. "She's praying for her child, and I am providing whatever medical resources are available to him. She is a very religious woman; she just did wonderfully." Holly says admiringly, "She's so strong. She had quite a bit of support by just believing that her child was going to survive. And he did." She adds laughing, "And he is wonderful."

"Today, this mother is heading an organization through the Internet, in contact with other parents, accessing the latest information by searching different hospital sites. She sometimes comes and tells me about some of the newest treatments." Holly appreciates having her share the information, admitting that as a pediatrician, she can't always keep up with the latest in cardiology or cardiac surgery.

Holly identifies three characteristics essential to being recognized as a good physician. The first is being professionally competent and keeping current in one's field. The second is being a down-to-earth type of person. Finally, third is being compassionate and holistic in one's approach to patients, guiding them through any pain and suffering.

She equates healing to caring for someone. As she says, "You may not be able to heal their disease, but you can care for them." Referring to the previously mentioned young, mentally disabled boy, she explains, "He comes into the office and this child does respond to my voice. Mom puts him on the exam table; he's now pretty big and well cared for. And then, I call his name, and he turns his head and smiles. This might be totally out of a reflex, but I think that he has been taken care of so beautifully by his mom, and maybe in part by me as a physician, that he has the ability to respond to a caring voice. Healing is such a powerful word; there is so much meaning to it."

Holly also concurs with one author's comment that he knows his patients want him to be a human being first and a physician second. "I get that from patients every day," she says nodding in agreement. "They want us to listen to them, and what they say is not always about their pain or their body parts. One of the things that I think that made my years of practice most satisfying involves providing the care that patients want or need."

Finally, to those young people contemplating a career in medicine, she advises, "I would say before making that decision, students should really be exposed to medicine to see how much they are willing to provide for another individual; how much they are willing to sacrifice. And if they are convinced that they can sacrifice more as a physician than in other professions, then they should apply to medical school."

Following His Bliss

W. F. (Dub) Howard, MD

Dub Howard is a reproductive endocrinologist with a large, successful practice in a rapidly growing Dallas Metroplex suburban community. He credits two early childhood experiences as key in guiding him toward medicine. "I was raised by very giving and very loving parents who themselves had great care for other people. They're not physicians, but they exhibited tremendous passion for their fellow man, for their friends, and for people they had never met before. So, I think that's number one," he says. With obvious love and gratitude, Dub considers his father his hero, who died at age 92, a short time after Linda sat down with Dub.

Second, he fondly remembers in the small east Texas town where he once lived, the physician who treated him occasionally. Dub remembers, "He had journals all over the place. He was always reading, always staying up to the minute on what was the latest in medicine. Of course, in those days," he chuckles, "there wasn't much new in medicine, but he was on top of whatever was available. Yet, you could go in and there was no rush. He would check my throat, or whatever, and then we would just sit and talk for a while. So, it was that feeling of rapport and closeness with that physician that really instilled in me what practicing medicine is all about."

Yet, Dub's path to medicine was indirect. Although he has practiced medicine for 30 years, he didn't become a physician until later in life. He recalls, "When I got to college, my intent was to go into chemistry or some scientific field." Medicine was not an option because in those days there weren't many scholarships available, and financial limitations caused him to discount that possibility. "I had some friends who were going to be pre-med students."

Although a part of him wished he was joining them in school, he scratched that off the list of possibilities because he believed he didn't have the resources. Eventually, he majored in counseling psychology, a field closely akin to his passion for helping people.

After a tour in the Air Force, he struggled over what to do next. "I was still very much at loose ends; I didn't know where I fit," he remembers. His inclination to build upon his degree led him to an encounter that would change his career direction. As he investigated graduate schools, his father referred him to a friend who was on the faculty of the psychology department at North Texas State University.

"I'll never forget it. The meeting took place at Howard Johnson's on Stemmons Freeway in Dallas. This was the only time I have ever seen this man in my life. He heard my story and my desire to work with people, to which he responded, 'Why don't you do it the right way. Go get your pre-med education and get a degree in psychiatry where you can treat the whole person.'"

"This is the true joy in life, the being used for a purpose recognized by yourself as a mighty one."

— George Bernard Shaw
Man and Superman (1905)

For Dub, it was like a light going on in his head. "It was sort of 'Me? Do you mean that?'" By then, Dub was 29. "By the time I went to bed that night, I had already laid my plans for what I was going to do." The University of Texas Southwestern Medical School reviewed his college transcript and outlined the courses required for admittance to medical school. He then enrolled in Southern Methodist University and subsequently was supported and encouraged by a number of faculty members who assisted him in gaining acceptance into medical school.

Dub Howard's career journey serves as a living testimony to James Hillman's theory, mentioned in the Introduction: some of us seem born with a vocational destiny. Dub's experiences, and especially the pivotal meeting at Howard Johnson's, also remind us of Joseph Jaworski's description of synchronicity. "We've all had those perfect moments, when things come together in an almost unbelievable way, when events that could never be predicted, let alone controlled, remarkably seem to guide us along the way."[5]

In *The Power of Myth*, Bill Moyers asks Joseph Campbell, "[Are we] being helped by hidden hands?" Campbell responds, "All the time. It is miraculous… if you do follow your bliss you put yourself on a kind of track that has been there all the while, waiting for

---

[5] Jaworski J. *Synchronicity: The Inner Path of Leadership.* San Francisco, CA: Berrett-Koehler; 1996: ix.

you, and the life you ought to be living is the one you are living."[6] Today, Dub continues to follow his bliss.

For Dub, passion means empathizing with another person's life and problems. It includes a willingness to work with them, either helping them directly or referring them to another resource.

"Passion is what my work is about. I've thought many times whether there was anything else I would rather be doing with my vocational life. I cannot think of anything else. I feel very blessed that I am being allowed to practice medicine. The idea of giving up my practice and removing myself from medicine is totally foreign to me. I have a patient who had two armed-forces tours of duty in Kosovo. She has shared with me some of the problems of the medical community in that area. The Serbs forced the Albanians from this area. The physicians were all removed from the hospital and were not allowed to practice for 10 years. For me, this would be a horrible event, being forced out of the field of medicine."

Asked what it means to be a good physician, Dub comments first about the importance of being a good listener in order to arrive at an understanding of the patient's problems. "First," he says, " I think a good doctor is one who listens to his or her patient. And, I am afraid that's a rare bird today, not because of lack of ability or training, but unfortunately with insurance being what it is, physicians are being forced to not listen but rather to do things as quickly as possible and not let the patient talk, because talking takes time. If you have been told by an insurance company that you have 8 minutes with a patient, total, then you can't sit and listen to that patient and hear out that person because they are not going to talk in Reader's Digest fashion. They're going to spill it out as they emote and as they feel and, therefore, that's not a quick thing. I think it's a tragedy. It's an art that is being lost," he says sadly.

"Most of my diagnoses are made by listening to what the patient tells me. Lab and technology simply confirm our suspicions. Ninety-five percent of the time the diagnosis is made before we ever go to the lab or to the operating room or anything else because the patient can tell you what's going on."

Dub believes that another characteristic of a good physician involves keeping current with medical literature—keeping on top of the conclusions of the medical experts in one's field. Dub

---

[6] Campbell J. *The Power of Myth*. New York, NY: Doubleday; 1988: 120.

feels strongly that good physicians know how to manage stress. "It must not be a hindrance to one's professional and personal life," he states emphatically.

Finally, a good physician will always admit when he or she simply does not know about a certain condition or the cause of an illness. "It is a matter of not letting pride get in your way and making stupid or false statements to the patient in order to make yourself sound smart. It is not an embarrassment to not know something," he says. For him, this also leads to a deeper appreciation of one's staff and the expertise of other health care professionals.

Dub's empathy for people, which is one of his key skills, has grown over the years. He has always seen himself as being a rather empathetic person, although this was eroded during his medical and postgraduate training at a county hospital in Texas where his approach to patients was typical for physicians at that hospital. They dealt with people in a less-than-human manner. "Often," he remembers, "there was no rapport whatsoever. It was like hitting a donkey with a two-by-four in order to get his attention and then whispering in his ear. The culture of that county hospital environment often necessitated abrasiveness," he says.

Then he moved to Utah for the second year of his residency and entered an environment very different from that of the county hospital. Soon thereafter, Dub received the wrath of his supervising physician for being abrupt. He attributes this experience as providing the foundation for his growth and maturity.

One of the hardest things Dub has done during his career is to give up his obstetrical work to concentrate on reproductive endocrinology. "That was hard," he admits, "because I enjoyed obstetrics." He laughs, "I didn't enjoy getting up at 3 o'clock in the morning; nobody does. But I never lost the joy and that thrill of delivering a baby. That was always exciting to me and always a neat thing to be a part of. But, it became very obvious if I was ever truly going to specialize in reproductive medicine, I had to give that up."

As often happens when patients are referred to a specialist, there is concern about the return of that patient to the referring practice. Although Dub always sent infertility patients back to their physicians, he believes the obstetricians were always thinking, "Am I going to lose that patient if I send her to Dub Howard?"

"And the other thing, of course," he adds, "was the fact that, from a psychological standpoint, it was terrible psychology for an infertility patient wanting to be pregnant so badly to sit out in the waiting room next to a 9-month OB [patient]. Also, I would be trapped over in labor and delivery for hours at a time waiting for a delivery while the infertility patients would be in the office waiting to be seen. They had to be seen that day because that was their cycle day; we had to do something, insemination or whatever. Therefore they couldn't come back another time. So, all of that put together just made it not feasible for me to continue to do OB."

Considering the current climate of health care and medicine today, Dub is both pessimistic and optimistic. "I have to be hopeful, because my heart won't let me be otherwise. But, what I see happening around me in medicine makes me feel very sad. Unfortunately, the bottom line rules today. The reason for it is corporate America and its influence upon the insurance industry. I hope that the people of this country will wake up eventually, and I think there are some signs of that occurring. We are even beginning to see anti-managed care themes being woven into the scripts of television programs."

Dub believes that America has the greatest medical system in the world, though others might not share this view. "Unfortunately, most of our citizens have no other system to compare it to in terms of quality." He underlines that, "We have no concept of what it means to have a gall bladder problem and to have to wait 6 months for surgery. It causes great stress for myself and for my colleagues to see us moving in this direction. We doctors don't think in terms of the bottom line. Our mission on this planet is to care for the health and welfare of our patients. My hope may be a false hope, but I want to work with managed care and still take care of the patient. I cannot give up."

Synergist of Heart and Mind

—Maile Anslinger, MD

We began our conversation with Dr Maile Anslinger by asking how it feels to cross the threshold from being a medical student to being a freshman MD, receiving her degree a few months earlier. She says, eyes sparkling, "In some ways it feels just terrific, the end of a lot of hard work. It's invigorating to take all of the learning and theory and instead of being told what to do, I am now able to make decisions myself. On the other hand," she adds gravely, "there is extra responsibility, a new weight, and now I have to give even more thought to my decisions."

Confessing that she is tired after a long day, Maile still exudes enthusiasm. The desire to make a difference in the lives of others led her into medicine. "I had it in my mind to enter medical school when I was a senior in college. Although," she quickly adds, "my sister claims that I had been talking about medicine for a long period of time. In any case, my love of science made the decision quite easy. During my college years, I also spent some time in Indonesia. It was certainly a different culture and, during this time, I gave a lot of thought to my career direction. I decided that caring for people meant helping them when they are most vulnerable."

For this book, we interviewed physicians who entered medicine over a wide span of years, representing a long continuum of health care. We were anxious to hear Maile's perceptions about entering the profession during this time of change and chaos. She believes people enter medicine for a number of reasons. "From experience with my colleagues fresh out of medical school, the strongest motivator seems to be service to others," she declares. "Even with all of the obstacles being placed in the way of doctors, it is still possible to provide for people's health needs. For example, the time we spend with each patient may be reduced to the point of not helping people with other problems in their lives, but I find it is still possible to have a therapeutic relationship. I also believe that people today enter medicine because they see it as a respected profession, even though that's not one of my stronger needs. And, even with reduced incomes these days, my salary will probably be more than my parents combined," she smiles. "I never wanted anything more than just to be comfortable."

"I think other young physicians have similar thoughts," she affirms. "I have had many conversations along these lines with one of my dearest friends from medical school, the thought being that we can use our brains and skills to help someone feel better. Also, I believe medical students today are being encouraged by others to think similarly."

"To write a prescription is easy, but to come to an understanding of people is hard."

— Franz Kafka
A Country Doctor (1916)

She recalls beginning her third clinical year. "I remember being encouraged to be a doctor who knows the patient most intimately, knowing the person beyond their medical history. In fact, we were encouraged to view the relationship as an opportunity to learn; patients can teach much of what we need to know about medicine. My professors used to say that patients may let their doctors into parts of their lives even hidden from family members."

"It's extraordinary to be allowed into such a sacred place," she says with some awe. "You can become very attached to these people. I take it hard when things don't go well and get very excited when they do. I understand that some distancing may be necessary for self-protection, but I've also seen many senior physicians who remain connected to their patients."

Knowing that physicians are not immune from their personal reaction to trauma and death, we were curious as to Maile's experiences in handling such trauma. "I remember almost every detail about my first experience," she recalls, sharing the story of a patient she met during her medicine rotation. "Diagnosed with HIV, this young man developed a life-threatening infection. I came to know him very well, spending a lot of time in conversation. He was very funny. He made jokes about everything. For example, he said the oncologist who took a bone marrow biopsy had the bedside manner of a street drunk," she laughs.

"The young man continued to get worse and eventually transferred to ICU, where I was not involved in his daily care. However, I continued to visit him, and was there about 2 hours before his family decided to remove the life support systems. I had an opportunity to say good-bye and to wish him peace wherever he might go after death. I cried all of the way home that day," she says with tears in her eyes, obviously still moved by the experience. As a student, she notes, "Few people ever spoke to me about such experiences. I did have a resident team leader address the subject of death. He told me that we always need to be prepared for these things. But essentially, it's something that I deal with on my own or with my family. My mother, my sister, and I are very close. I find comfort in speaking to them about trauma and death."

Maile reports that as a student, she did participate in a remarkable 2-day course on death and dying, part of her introduction to clinical medicine. Lectures and panel discussions provided a great deal of information on the subject. A hospice representative spoke about that program. Chaplains and social workers also talked about transitioning to compassionate care and about end-of-life issues. Some of the panels included classmates describing the losses they had suffered in their lives. "That was a very moving part of the course, and a lot of the participants ended up in tears."

"We also discussed some of the ethical issues surrounding end-of-life occurrences. What is important to the patient? What does he or she want to have happen? Whom do they want making decisions? So we did have some preparation as medical students, but I am not sure there is any way to prepare for how you feel when losing a patient."

Continuing, Maile remembers, "There was a psychiatrist who visited one of our courses during the second year of medical school. At the beginning of her talk, she said that as students we will feel very connected to our patients and we will care about them. She asked us never to lose such relationships and feelings. It's the old Francis Peabody quotation: 'The secret to caring for the patient is caring for the patient.'"

"[The doctor] brings air and cheer into a sick room, and often enough, though not so often as he wishes, brings healing."

— Robert Louis Stevenson
Preface to *Underwoods* (1887)

Maile views medicine as her passion. For her, passion is something that absorbs a person, commanding the heart and mind. "Even during tough days I love what I do," she says excitedly. "It's so challenging, sometimes painfully so, but most of the time in a stimulating way. I get to use my brain all of the time and work out problems. It's always different and exciting. You think about ways to help a patient. Sometimes treatments work and sometimes they don't, but it's always so interesting. You find yourself dealing with the complexities of both medicine and people. Just in terms of dealing with people," she grins, "you experience so much variety; they can be funny, pleasant, interesting, anxious, or grumpy. It's neat to be able to speak with them and make a difference in their lives. I think of my work more as a privilege than anything else. I feel so lucky that I have the skills for this profession. I really don't know what else I could do vocationally that would have as much meaning as medicine."

Maile shared a recent evaluation of her medical skills that included self-perceptions of her nontechnical expertise. Key among those nonclinical proficiencies is being able to communicate and help her patients better understand what is happening to them, explaining things clearly and teaching people what she knows. As she states, "During my first year in medical school, I remember listening to a clinical medicine professor who had been practicing for 50 years. He said the derivation of the word 'doctor' comes from the word 'teacher.' I take this seriously, explaining the 'what and why' of a person's condition. We can do so much more for people if they understand what is happening, and if they care about it. I've done a lot of teaching over the years unrelated to medicine, so I see it as a primary talent of mine."

Maile finds it almost easier for a woman than a man to be a physician these days, suggesting that a woman is almost expected to be more nurturing. Stereotyping exists, of course, but being a female physician allows her to show her caring. Sometimes physicians are expected to be rather impersonal and aloof, perhaps because there are so many specialists who see patients for a limited period of time. However, she states, "If I cry with a family over a difficult situation, it doesn't make me seen as being weak, which may not be true for a man."

"When it comes to lifestyle issues, being a woman can make it harder," she acknowledges. "You have to decide whether to get married, have children, and expand your various roles. Many of my female colleagues who are married receive considerable financial support from their spouses, so there is room for give and take. Also, there are expanding opportunities available today such as working part time or job sharing."

Both spirit and prayer are important for Maile in her perceptions of caring for her patients and in health care in general. Coincidentally, she tells us, "We were just talking about that today, although that is unusual. With some patients it seems appropriate to discuss spiritual issues, and it is important to be open about it. It's part of accepting a patient's situation and needs, and it's often a part of the 'why' question, as in 'why is this happening to me?' I attempt to explain that there are other forces at work in healing or not-healing processes that remain beyond our understanding. We have no control over them, at least not to our knowledge."

Quietly, she says, "I have prayed with a patient; you never know what might happen because of it. It could be that a patient heals because she or he believes in the power of prayer, or perhaps it works in some other, mysterious way. In any case, peacefulness emerges when I pray with someone. Some kind of connection occurs. It can also contribute to making peace with the potential end of life."

Maile views healing and curing as not being synonymous, believing that healing addresses the person as a whole as opposed to a particular disease. "When we are involved in healing we are ministering to the mind and soul of a person as well as the body," she says intently. "When I am on my morning rounds speaking with patients, I constantly remind myself that I am not here just for the purpose of tending to an illness. For example, if someone states that he or she is scared about a particular procedure, we talk about that and I make sure they understand what will happen. That's all part of the healing process. I'm not simply a pill-pusher."

"That's why I believe the power of healing really resides in the relationship between doctor and patient. It builds upon the passion and compassion of the physician, and upon the trust of the patient. If the patient doesn't trust you, then all of the technology and interventions will have a limited impact. Sometimes the interventions don't work, but healing occurs anyway because of the power of trust. Healing comes from the integration of heart and mind in both the doctor and the patient."

Maile's decision to specialize in internal medicine came about, in part, because of her internal medicine rotation as a student. Practically from the start of the rotation she had an "ah ha," she tells us enthusiastically. She likes the diversity, as well as the opportunity to be a primary care physician.

Where she ultimately practices is also important. "I like the idea of living in a smaller community," she admits. "I grew up in a small Alaska town. Also, my parents are just now retiring and moving to a warmer, sunnier climate; I might move closer to them."

Decidedly, she sees herself being part of a group practice. "Ideally, I will practice with a small group of other internists in which each person has a special interest. For example, I'm very interested in infectious disease; someone else in the practice may have additional training in cardiology. In any case, I think it is important to have colleagues. Being able to work out problems in a group is very important. I did a 6-month rotation in family medicine in a little town in Wyoming. I was the only medical student for many miles, so it wasn't possible to share experiences with my peers. It caused me to realize how important it is to be part of a team."

Admittedly very optimistic about the future of health care, she recognizes the current system's irritants, including the frustrations that come when insurance companies give directives. Maile concedes that she can be as frustrated as anyone else.

"On the other hand," she asserts, "there are a lot of things in life that are frustrating. But it's not the end-all be-all. My mother always used to say, 'This too shall pass,'" she says grinning at the memory. "The pendulum swings back and forth. The opportunities are always present to make connections with patients and reaffirm why we became doctors in the first place. Even the gloom-and-doom predictions don't seem that bad to me. I shrug my shoulders and move on."

Concluding our interview, she says seriously, "Some of the pessimism in medicine comes from unrealistic expectations. Personally, I don't really expect much in terms of monetary compensation. I don't expect the paperwork to recede. [Gloomy] predictions don't bother me because I have high expectations only for myself in terms of serving my patients."

And, though the day has already been a long one, she leaves us to complete her rounds before calling it a day.

Living the Three I's of Passion

Sanjiv Parikh, MD

One letter Dr Sanjiv Parikh received reads,

"Dear Dr Parikh: I want to thank you for your steady hand on Tuesday when you performed my biopsy. I have had others quite a bit more painful. I also want you to know I appreciated you allowing my wife to observe. I know it raised your level of discomfort, but it allowed us to continue to face each step together. This may seem strange to you, but since we have been married we've faced everything together—her masters degree, her mother's death, my struggle with terminal cancer—we've faced it together. Your increased tension was the price of allowing us to continue to walk this out together. You will possibly never know how much we appreciated your going against established procedures, but it helped us a great deal."

As one might assume, most radiologists do not receive letters of appreciation from patients. But for Sanjiv, director of interventional radiology at Seattle's Swedish Providence campus, such letters are not unusual. As an interventional radiologist, he brings what he calls the "three I's of passion" to his practice: *intensity, integrity,* and *inner enthusiasm.* "Together, they serve as a joy and passion, something I intensely love and cherish," he explains.

Such passion often distinguishes an outstanding physician from a mediocre one and can be witnessed in the way Sanjiv practices medicine. "Obviously you must be a good diagnostician and good in your specialty, always attempting to improve yourself," he affirms. "But most importantly, it involves having a caring and compassionate relationship with a patient. You make a sincere effort to understand and empathize with the person and the problem. A good doctor actively listens, makes good eye contact, and is able to look at what's behind the immediate situation confronting him or her. When you listen with your heart, it touches patients."

As any number of physicians can testify, the pathway to passion is not always straightforward. For the first 25 years of his life, Sanjiv lived in India where his dream to become a physician first surfaced as a young boy. "Actually," he recalls, "I can track it back to elementary school. It was triggered by a couple of things. My uncle is a very well-known surgeon in India. During summer vacation visits, he would take me to his hospital operating room showing me his work. I realized early on that I was not fazed by blood or serious illnesses. It was very interesting to me. Although at that point I didn't realize it, the sick people I saw along the roads also impacted me; they simply looked ill and I never understood why. I thought if I became a doctor, I could figure it out. As you know, TB, malaria, and malnutrition represent fairly common, day-to-day problems in India. Solving them became an inspiration for me. Every year when I went to visit my uncle, it became clearer I wanted to be a doctor. By eighth grade, I began working toward that goal."

However, Sanjiv's original desire to become a surgeon never materialized. "It is very hard to get into medical school in India," he relates. "The odds are one in a hundred, and then, only the top few people in the class would be able to train for surgery." He managed to get into medical school but failed the next cut. "I was disappointed, but worked through the setback, exploring ways to get close to surgery. In India at that time, interventional radiology was just becoming a field of study, the next best thing to surgical treatment. After my training, I decided to come to the US for more education with the very clear goal of becoming an interventional radiologist in the States."

Continuing, he recalls, "As a foreign medical school graduate, it was very difficult to get into residency training in radiology. I started with clinical research, published papers, sat through arduous tests (I do not test very well on K-type questions), and finally got accepted to Northwestern University for postgraduate training. After 8 years, I finished my postgraduate training in nuclear medicine, diagnostic radiology, and interventional radiology."

Interventional radiology differs from the field of radiology in major ways, notes Sanjiv. A diagnostic radiologist typically focuses on reading and interpreting X rays, ultrasound, CAT scans, MRIs, and so on, while the focus of an interventional radiologist is different. He or she utilizes these diagnostic modalities for treatment purposes. These treatments are performed usually under local anesthesia, utilizing very small incisions of less than 3 millimeters. And, unlike the diagnostic radiologist, the interventionalist does visit patients.

Although becoming a surgeon was his original dream, Sanjiv reports, "My current work has become my passion. During my training, I was fortunate to be exposed to fascinating radiological interventions. I had excellent mentors during my residency program. I nurtured the love I had for the profession, and I did additional fellowship training in this field. Interventional radiology is now a board-certified subspecialty, following radiology training. I have been able to further expand my horizon, working with a well-known vascular surgeon, Dr Kaj Johansen, and developing new techniques in the field."

Sanjiv's current facility is reputed to have the largest program treating narrowed or blocked arteries going to the stomach and small bowel. "It's truly been very much a passion for me beyond me just treating the patient," he again affirms.

Sanjiv believes understanding the role of soul in medicine enhances the patient–physician relationship and directly impacts how a patient is perceived. "Most physicians hone in on the physical aspects of sickness or disease in patients," he declares. "Soul in medicine relates to how, as a human being, the physician's social, cultural, and emotional makeup interacts with the patient's body, mind, and spirit."

"Ultimately it is the physician's respect for the human soul that determines the worth of his science."

— Norman Cousins
Anatomy of an Illness (1979)

Along with others, he believes there is a resurgence of interest in enhancing the soul of physicians. "It always intrigued me why this aspect of medicine was never stressed in medical school," he quizzes. "I didn't hear anyone speaking about it. We didn't really get any practical pointers during training or residency. It was kind of hit and miss in terms of experiencing an emotional reaction to one patient, then using it during the next encounter. I think when physicians come together and begin talking about soul, it will be very beneficial for them and for future doctors."

Reflecting upon the power of healing, Sanjiv asserts, "I simply feel I am an instrument of God. I have been trained in the science of taking care of patients, but I truly believe that we as physicians are instruments of some higher power. The positive energy to treat a patient comes from within and beyond us."

"The typical patient coming to me has problems related to the narrowing of vessels. Their quality of life is impacted by the inability to walk or their bad hypertension. With this type of patient, a very high probability exists we will be able to impact a cure. However, a patient's hope is also quite important. When a patient comes to the physician, he or she enters not simply with a particular problem, but with the emotional impact the problem has had upon their quality of life. I'm not saying that we can paint a rosy picture all the time, but giving patients realistic hope and striving to actualize it, well, that's what makes a good doctor."

Sanjiv also believes spirit and prayer play very important roles in healing. "As a matter of fact," he affirms, "at least to some degree, it has been substantially shown that, when both patient and doctor engage in practices of the spirit, the likelihood of success accelerates." He offers meditation as an example. "When I am doing a procedure, I get into a meditative rhythm while dealing with the task at hand or the disease process. In my mind, integrating your spirit and soul while the procedure takes place makes a huge difference. We deal with very delicate structures, sometimes very complex situations. Meditative concentration helps a great deal. One of my mentors, Dr Nemcek, at Northwestern University, used to say, 'when you approach an artery, you, the needle, and the artery become one.' I truly believe that."

"God is a sphere whose center is everywhere and whose circumference is nowhere."

— Gnostic Proverb

As an example where a procedural outcome was unexpectedly positive, Sanjiv shares this story. "I will never forget a 41-year-old lady who came into the ER with severe vaginal bleeding. Religious concerns prevented a blood transfusion. She was a chronic alcoholic and had previous bleeding episodes, but this was a very severe one. She was admitted to the ICU and, for the most part, everyone had given up hope because her platelet, hemoglobin, and hematocrit levels were so low. None of the surgeons wanted to touch her, and I was consulted as a last resort. After talking with the doctors involved in her care and with her mother, I knew there was very little chance of saving her. I expressed a realistic hope that we might be able to salvage the situation, but by the same token she might die on the table. Her mother accepted the risks involving the procedure, primarily because there weren't many options left."

"I remember it was a very busy day, but I could sense a strong, inner drive to treat her. Fortunately everything happened according to plan and we hardly lost any blood during the procedure. We were also able to suture her artery after we stopped the bleeding from her uterus. She stabilized that night and when I went to visit her the next morning. I was shocked by the fact she was doing so much better. Here was a situation most of the physicians thought hopeless, but she got progressively better, her blood values started to improve significantly, and she was actually discharged in about 4 days after the procedure. About 6 weeks later, she underwent an uneventful, elective hysterectomy. There are quite a few of these situations in my practice, but this sticks out as being really high on the list. That's why I feel there is something beyond you and me, and why it makes me feel like an instrument."

It is easy to view Sanjiv's three "I's" of passionate enthusiasm reflected in his work. They greatly influence his view of medicine. They also impact why he is cautiously optimistic about the future of medicine. He says, "I think physicians, practicing today and in the future, have significant stress and hardships on a day-to-day basis. Having said this, I think if we can rekindle the soul of the physician, then he or she will be able to look at these problems from a different perspective and will not let them affect the core of the doctor–patient relationship."

"Recently a young man considering a medical career came seeking my advice. Here's what I had to tell him," Sanjiv explains. "I first asked him, 'Why medicine?' When I found he was not very sure about his reasons, I gave him my side of the story. I told him there are probably many ways of making a good living nowadays, very enticing careers like investment banking, securities advisor, or a dot-com entrepreneur. Medicine may be a financially rewarding profession, but the real rewards will not be in the form of money. They come from passion for the profession. I told him about my passion of coming to work on a day-to-day basis, even in the midst of all the difficulties. I had to admit that things are getting harder and harder. Having to deal with insurance companies, lawyers, and others are all part of being a doctor these days. You also have to deal with failures in your work. I gave him a realistic picture based upon my experience. I think it is a terrific profession, but you must rise above a lot of issues and not let them decrease your enthusiasm to take care of people."

Continuing, he amplifies, "One of the reasons people used to choose medicine as a profession was security. That meant having a job and making a reasonable living. On both those counts today, there exists a fair amount of uncertainty." Nonetheless, Sanjiv has no plans to pursue another vocational avenue in the future.

He states enthusiastically, "I love what I do. I am pretty sure there will be a place for me to practice, if not here, somewhere else. I will just go on and make it happen. I cherish teaching as well as clinical research. Those may be some avenues I may nurture, but I don't think I will ever give up my clinical practice. Today, I teach at the university and at the hospital. I'm also involved in a fair amount of lecturing locally and nationally."

Sanjiv's favorite quote is in Sanskrit and he translates its meaning into English. "It basically means that you have the right to action and it's within you to take that action, but you do not have the right to the fruit of the action. In short, keep doing good work; rewards may or may not come." And then he adds laughing heartily, "Lately, they don't come."

REFORMERS/ACTIVISTS

"After decades of crisis, medicine wants to renew itself as
a healing art. It wants to nourish patients and free them
from the haunting malady of meaninglessness."
—Deepak Chopra, MD

Being on Call

Todd Pearson, MD

If and when Dr Todd Pearson writes a book, it might be titled *Being On Call, Authentic Presence, Spirit in Action, and the Courage to Care*. It would be about "being" in the sense of Shakespeare's assertion, "To be or not to be." Todd states, "It involves investing in our inner selves. It would not be about 'doing,' because our doing naturally manifests from the cultivation of our being. 'On call' means paying attention to all of the clues every day, internally and externally, that would help us to develop and cultivate our true sense of identity and purpose on earth. The very nature of being on call is about authentic presence, spirit, courage, and compassion in action."

No specific instances drew Todd toward medicine. His decision was powered by many early childhood experiences.

"I came from a very dysfunctional family. My parents divorced when I was very young and Mom left the family, so I had abandonment issues to deal with. My father even attempted to commit suicide, so I had to grow up real quickly. I believe that many people who enter the helping and healing professions do so because of an early childhood wounding. It becomes a form of compensation for what was lacking. It's a kind of zealous overcompensation for what was missing in early life experiences."

"Looking at some of the wisdom traditions, it's not atypical for people to transform life's tragedies of pain and suffering into a vocation requiring compassion. I believe that a number of physicians would describe their early childhood as dysfunctional."

And yet in spite of such family dysfunction, Todd reports that at some point during his childhood he was given unconditional, positive regard. Someone gave him a message that he could achieve just about any goal he set for his life. Reflecting upon it, he declares, "Aside from a large amount of self-cultivation, I probably received this [positive regard] from a woman who came into my life during pre-adolescent and adolescence years. She dated my father for a period of time and continues to be a surrogate mother to me. She became the first person who gave me an awareness of what safe space is all about, a sanctuary and refuge where you can remember who you are, what is important, and why you are here on earth. She ended up being my mentor, surrogate mother, and confidant."

Todd attended medical school at Oregon's Health Sciences Center and completed his residency at Children's Hospital and at the University of Washington in Seattle. He chose pediatrics because it related back to his childhood and to a natural inclination to help kids. Also, he was drawn to this specialty because of his experiences during his medical school clerkships. He says, "For the most part, the residents in this specialty seemed to have a sense of life/family/work balance and priorities. All through medical school, I attempted to maintain that sense of balance."

> "The best parts of a good man's life are those little, nameless, unremembered acts of kindness and love."
>
> —William Wordsworth
> (1798)

"In fact, I had real struggles with the whole idea of entering medical school. I knew there was great potential for losing my sense of self. I didn't open up my letter of acceptance for 2 weeks as it lay in the glove compartment of my old VW bug. It was a thin envelope and the belief at the time was that if you received such an envelope, it meant a rejection. To this day, I don't know if I delayed opening this letter because I was afraid of rejection or because I was afraid of acceptance. Heavily into mountain climbing and investing in my personal growth, I took 2 years off between college and medical school. I knew deep inside what it would mean if I were accepted. There would be whole parts of myself disavowed and lost. So I was petrified about what entering medicine would mean."

During his years as a practicing pediatrician, Todd maintained a passion for the profession, more so with relationships than with technical knowledge and competence in technique. What meant the most to him in his practice remains foremost in his values today. However, through the years these relationships to himself, to significant others, and to patients became increasingly compromised, contributing to his vacillating feelings of being in and out of burnout.

In 1994, Todd decided to take a 3-month sabbatical from his very successful pediatric practice. As shared in our first book, "he immersed himself in books from very diverse fields, including self-help, spirituality, career development, leadership, and many others. He totally invested in himself, something he had never really done before, at least not with this level of intensity."

During his sabbatical, he became curious about what resources might be available for health care professionals such as himself.

He knew that he was not the only person suffering in silence. In the Northwest, there were some career counselors whose general practice included physicians, but they were not in touch with the issues and concerns of the medical profession. Todd expanded his search nationally and began to network, seeking resources specifically geared to physicians. His search became an all-consuming passion, the answer to his personal "Why?" and became much more of a calling for him than medicine had been. During this period, he developed a vision of a center where physicians could come for renewal, a place that would address their multiple human resource concerns.[1] So, in 1996, he opened The Center for Physician Renewal in the Seattle area.

Today, his passion expands to the healing of health care, including its individual, organizational, and cultural transformation. With great enthusiasm, he asserts, "I am passionate about the creation of a movement mentality within health care that is relationship centered, helping to transform its culture, the profession, and the very nature of service that it provides. I am passionate about grassroots social activism rooted in spirituality. In fact, I increasingly witness it happening and I can't help but be optimistic about the trends as they keep showing up in my work. It shows up in my clients, in participants during retreats and seminars I facilitate, and in attendees at conferences in which I am asked to do keynote presentations. I believe in the principles of synchronicity and the laws of attraction as I see people come forth who are also passionate about health care reform and transformation."

"This passion springs not only from an intellectual expression, but people want to take the next step toward embodying transformation in their personal lives. To use Parker Palmer's model, these are people who are no longer willing to live and work a divided life.[2] They are making a very personal, deep decision that they can no longer do this and are finding a new center for the ground of their being. To put it another way, the process of transformation cannot unfold using the logic of our health care organizations or the logic of medicine's mainstream culture at large, but it's finding one's personal meaning in the depths of one's life. It doesn't mean they are leaving medicine or even the

---

[1] Henry LG, Henry JD. *Reclaiming Soul in Health Care: Practical Strategies for Revitalizing Providers of Care.* Chicago, IL: AMA Press; 1999: 77–78.
[2] Palmer PJ. *Let Your Life Speak, Listening for the Voice of Vocation.* San Francisco, CA: Jossey-Bass; 1999.

organization in which they work, but they are operating from a very different place. A shift in consciousness occurs, a shift in how they see themselves, relationships, and how they see the world of health care."

Todd continues, "Having initiated this shift, these people are naturally attracted to other individuals who have made the same inward decision, forming a subculture or communities of congruence. They essentially create a refuge or sanctuary to practice these ways of being, of seeing, and believing. They then summon up a common courage to go back into the workplace and embody this new way of living in the world. At some point, this includes going public with their perceptions, converting their private concerns into the public issues they indeed are."

Given the current health care climate, we wondered how such physicians survive. How can one make such a deep personal and sacred commitment to the integrity of relationships with oneself and others, yet at the same time remain in what many describe as an increasingly assembly-line medicine model?

Todd reports, "Most of them remain in their current practices and organizations. It's not a matter of leaving medicine, nor do they change the particulars of their work. Rather, they change their experience of work and how they view themselves. They transform how they view their relationship to constraints, control, change, risk, and to power and to where, in fact, power lies within the world of health care. All of this shifts and in the process, they move past their sense of disconnection and transcend their own fears. And in so doing, they move toward relationship."

Todd suggests that these physicians view managed care as a painful stage in the process of healing and transforming our health care system. "They remember why they are present and whom and what they are serving. They are keenly aware of their motivations and innate skills. They offer their best professional service in the midst of the constraints. The issue is one of fidelity. It involves fidelity to who they most essentially are as a healer, and to what's important to them and why they are here. And, it includes fidelity to these same matters in the patient who sits across from them in the exam room. They no longer portray an onstage appearance disconnected from their essential nature. More fascinating, it ends up evoking the same stance in the patient."

Todd believes that there are many instances within health care of how a movement mentality can help transform our health care system. Many of these models have converged methodologies from both the social movements and the consciousness movements that have existed in our country over the last four decades. Both the hospice and palliative care movements and the integrative medicine-holistic health movements are good examples. Through both direct personal action and internal shifts, individuals change their worldview, way of living (and dying), and way of working. They come together with kindred spirits who share similar beliefs and values and begin to challenge the mainstream cultural codes, educate "moral" publics, and change the (spoken/unspoken) rules and paradigms. In some cases, they may successfully challenge the conventional political, economic, and health care establishments and actually create a change in policies and actions in the external world.

For many people, entering such a transformational journey requires great courage. In *The Hero with a Thousand Faces*, Joseph Campbell describes it as entering a "wasteland," facing how one has lived an inauthentic life. Some may choose the journey, while others remain petrified by fear, anxiety, and the dread of being ostracized by family, friends, or peers.[3] We wondered about what happens in the life of a physician motivating him or her to embark on such a path.

"It's not unique to medicine," Todd replies. "It's part of the human condition. What events cause us to enter such a transition? It might be pain and suffering, either our own in terms of a health challenge or just the fact that you experience a drastic disconnection from your sense of calling. At some point, you say to yourself and others, 'I can't do it this way anymore.'"

"On the other hand, it may be having a vision of some kind. You have this image of something you want to create and it pulls you forward. It may be both a disconnect and a vision, like four-wheel drive on a car. The pain and suffering pushes from behind while at the same time a gravitational force pulls you forward. Pain and vision can both melt fear."

Todd's insights remind us of a formula offered by career counselor Dr Helen Harkness in her book, *The Career Chase*.

"CC = P > F [indicates] that career change takes place only when the pain of the current situation is greater than the fear of the unknown and of the potential new situation." [4]

---

[3] Campbell J. *The Hero with a Thousand Faces*. Princeton, NJ: Princeton University Press; 1949.

[4] Harkness H. *The Career Chase*. Palo Alto, CA: Davies-Black Publishing; 1996: xv.

We might alter the equation to CC = V + P > F, incorporating the tremendous energy of having a vision in the change process.

Todd received certification as a senior coach in individual and organizational coaching with the Hudson Institute of Santa Barbara. We asked him to describe how he applies particular tools and processes in helping physicians move toward transformation.

"One can live magnificently in this world if one knows how to work and how to love, to work for the person one loves, and love one's work."

—Leo Tolstoy

He replies, "I would have answered your question quite differently as a practicing physician. I would have thought about what tools and techniques could be applied to the healing of people. How am I going to help and fix someone, as if I am the one with the power to help a person change for the better? Today, I am in a totally different place. When I am interviewed by medical publications writing articles about medical burnout, they want to know where I am headed when I meet with a client and what needs to be done. My answer is that I have a commitment to the process and I am not attached to the outcomes or some specific result. I pay attention to what is emerging in our relationship, to what has heart and meaning in the moment. Where we end up at the end of the relationship often is quite a surprise."

He continues, "A client may come to me and say that all he can tell me is what he doesn't like about his work. He or she confides their possibility of leaving medicine altogether. I'll affirm this as a possibility, but I'm not attached to that outcome. Overwhelmingly as we have integrity to the journey, I don't use tools or assessments; rather, I create a space. If I truly listen, then perhaps clients begin to listen to themselves as well. They begin to remember who they are and what is important in their lives, that personal 'why.' They may hear their own story for the first time."

"Essentially, I do two things. First, I bear witness by genuinely listening to their story. Secondly, I walk with them. The analogy is that I walk with them for a little way on their journey home. I may plant some seed thoughts, exercises, or questions. Then they live the questions as though the questions were their companions. There is not necessarily a single answer or a right–wrong answer or a final answer, but they begin to hold the questions as a practice in mindfulness. The issues may be around congruency or authenticity; how someone may be out of harmony with who he or she is. I do this in a nonjudgmental or nonevaluative manner. So, I would say what I most essentially do is to create safe space."

Todd describes the essence of the coach–client relationship as one of sharing stories, arriving at the reality that what is most personal is also most universal. It's about listening and not about fixing someone. It's about compassion, and he subscribes to the overflow theory of compassion. Before someone can practice compassion, they must fill themselves up first. He says, "When I speak about social activism in transforming health care, the place to begin is through self-awareness, self-care, and self-compassion. If these are practiced, compassion for others simply, naturally shows up."

Todd suggests that one of the vital, ongoing challenges involves transcending cultural shadow, the often dark, unconscious collective beliefs and behaviors of a group or society. He asserts that, "In health care, cultural shadow requires examining our education and training as physicians. The root word for education is 'educare,' meaning to lead forth toward wholeness. My medical education was just the opposite; it was indoctrination. In the course of attending medical school, we must disavow whole parts of ourselves for the purpose of acceptance and approval. Cultural shadow serves as a collective, underground belief system wounding the spirit of a person through judgment."

"For example, consider the opposite polarities of *objective* and *subjective*. We are rewarded in health care if we disconnect from our subjective self. Objectivity and professionalism receive the reward. People in health care who are being held in the highest regard, who are seen externally as being the most successful, very often embody the deepest cultural wound. They remain disconnected from their subjective, feeling self in favor of objectivity. Mastery reigns over mystery and control sways over surrender. Measurable outcomes and tangible results become all important; anything that cannot be quantified or explained is held at arms length. Truth that cannot be objectified somehow becomes threatening."

Continuing, he says, "In the culture of physicianhood, being vulnerable and suffering in the process of caring for patients is seen as a sign of weakness. So our own liabilities, limitations, and inadequacies recede into one's unconscious shadow. Yet, in many ways, facing our pain and liabilities sets the stage for the beginning of compassion. In addition, there are incredible innate gifts and talents available to physicians that are disavowed because they are not encouraged and reinforced in the health care system. These qualities of being and relationship and these innate gifts could hugely impact the patient encounter, as well as relationships between colleagues. Just think about how it would change the quality of health care if we could bring our total, compassionate selves to the environment without wearing masks."

Todd is deeply passionate about relationship-centered care. He is a co-coordinator of the relationship-centered care movement supported by the Fetzer Institute and is starting a Northwest regional network. Currently, there are about 300 people across the United States who exhibit passion about the subject and are part of the movement. The relationship-centered care movement values and embraces the well-being of the practitioner, the patient, and our public and professional communities and looks at relationships existing between all of the stakeholders in health care.

People involved in the transformational movement come from all areas of health care including insurance companies and public policy groups. They also include patients, administrators, and practitioners who come from different disciplines, traditions, and practices in both conventional, allopathic medicine and from complementary and alternative health care. Todd affirms, "Many of them are passionate about bringing soul and spirituality to health care. They desire to bring spirituality into our relationships and our work."

Exploring this a little deeper, we asked Todd to share his concept of soul and spirit. He addressed the subject at two levels.

"I'm a pilgrim when it comes to this subject, so I don't claim to have expertise," he cautions. "Often, we teach what we need to learn. But, part of soul simply involves the innate capacity we all have for spiritual experience. The other part reflects a state of being. The analogies and synonyms coming to mind include authentic self, divine self, God self, and true self. Soul is the life force residing within us, through which spirit is present. Soul manifests itself when we are actually able to embody that energy. Soul is not an idea or an intellectual library in the head, but a dynamism coming into play when we get it out of the head. People who are able to do this narrow the gap between having an intellectual awareness and walking the talk. In its purest sense, perhaps soul is unadulterated awareness."

Todd believes that connecting to soul begins with a relationship to oneself, then to others with a kind of ripple effect. Finally, we connect to some phenomenon, name it as you like, that is much larger than what we can conceive.

Because of his deep commitment to spirit and soulful healing, people often wonder why Todd left medicine. That seems quite bizarre to him, because today he sees himself as more intimately involved in the profession than ever before.

He relates, "When I was a practicing pediatrician, I became lost among the trees in the forest. I had an incredibly busy practice, seeing patients and teaching on the staff of several hospitals and on all kinds of different committees. However, today I am so much closer to the big picture of health care. I can see the forest, the trees, and the territory ahead. I am more *in* medicine than ever before."

The key to Todd's authentic involvement in health care relates to taking care of himself first. "I exercise, meditate, read extensively, nourish my inner life, and spend a lot of time in nature. I am also a part of a community of congruence. It is so important to be connected to other individuals who share my values."

"But most importantly, taking care of oneself involves the lifelong process of wrestling with cultural shadow. Cultural shadow is much different than family shadow," he claims. "Family shadow is fairly unique and there are many people and resources to help us overcome its dysfunctional energies. But cultural shadow transcends time and geography. It's very pervasive, showing up in almost every social interaction. It calls us to conformity and we are really never finished overcoming it. So, in doing my own inner work and in serving my clients, it becomes a matter of transforming how we see ourselves and how we see the world. We are able to look at how we relate to such things as risk, reward, consequences, control, and power. It involves a change of consciousness."

"So, we begin with ourselves. If you think the problem is outside of yourself, then that is the problem. So you ask yourself, how have I been a part of the silent conspiracy? How have I kept myself in denial and, in so doing, have kept myself stuck? How have I contributed to the dehumanization of health care? These are the kinds of questions that we in the profession must continue to live with. On the other hand, we must continually explore and reclaim our innate human skills and talents, utilizing them in the service of others."

In summary, Todd asserts that most people engage in a movement like relationship-centered care because they love the profession. They love their practice and the institution of medicine, not wanting to see it stoop to its lowest form. They work to transform anger and cynicism. In *The Art of Possibility*, Rosamund and Benjamin Zander describe a cynic as "a person who does not want to be disappointed again." [5] The authors suggest that to address such a person is not to speak to the cynicism but to speak to his/her passion. Building on this, Todd suggests, "There is a form of anger rooted in love as opposed to hate, indifference, and judgment. So it's a matter of taking negative energy aimed at the current health care system and converting it to more constructive and helpful ends."

[5] Zander R, Zander B. *The Art of Possibility*. Boston, MA: Harvard Business School Press; 2000: 39.

Medical and Social Activist

Roy G. Farrell, MD

We began our interview with Dr Roy Farrell, chief of emergency services, Group Health Cooperative, Seattle, by asking him about his understanding of the word *soul*. Our discussion led to an exploration of his passionate activities within and beyond medicine. Roy describes *soul* as "the very essence of who we are." His very clear understanding of this essence is that we are spiritual beings who happen to be embodied in flesh and that we are children of God along with all of our fellow human beings.

Roy agrees with the mystic Matthew Fox, who states in his book, *Original Blessing*,[6] that the starting point for our basic self-understanding is the goodness as described in the first chapter of Genesis. "And God saw everything that he made, and behold, it was very good."

Roy says, "This doesn't mean that we don't make mistakes, but at our core we are holy, spiritual beings. When I am in touch with my soul I am in touch with a deep connection with the universal life energy and with the earth."

> "We walk through forests of physical things that are also spiritual things that look on us with affectionate looks."
>
> —Charles Baudelaire
> The Flower of Evil (1857)

"Medicine is such a wonderful career because we are dealing with this life force in a much more direct way than many other people are able to do. I believe that, in the final analysis, every interaction is spiritual in nature, as is every calling and every career, but in medicine the spiritual connection is so much closer to the surface. This spiritual connection is a great part of the inherent reward I get from being a physician. It involves touching the whole person in ways that are special and privileged. In this respect, hopefully the doctor–patient relationship is rewarding to both of us."

As with most of the physicians we interviewed, Roy describes his work as his passion. "Passion is that enthusiasm that we feel for our work and other activities. It involves a sense that you are good at what you do and can make a difference. Even though we

---

[6] Fox M. *Original Blessing*. Santa Fe, NM: Bear & Co; 1983.

might be exposed to stressful and even tragic situations, passion includes the gratitude you feel in being able to help people through their difficulty. It involves a respectful thankfulness that you are able to service in this role."

However, he states that his is a balanced passion. "I don't give everything I have to give at the office or the hospital. As an emergency physician, I also do a lot of things outside of my job that give me extreme pleasure. For example, I am on the board of directors for the Physicians for Social Responsibility."

He knows that it might be easier for him to achieve balance than for many other physicians because of his work in the emergency department. He may work four shifts during the week, but knows that he will have 3 additional days to put his energies into other activities.

"Can it be that one of the greatest obstacles to world citizenship today is the lack of awareness that the ideal is not only possible, but mandatory?"

—Norman Cousins

"My community-related activities have been very important to me. I was very active in citizen diplomacy in the old Soviet Union, attempting to figure out whom these people were that Ronald Reagan was calling the 'evil empire.' It appeared that he wanted to bomb them off the face the earth. I was a part of the first physician exchange between two sister cities in the US and the Soviet Union. Many of the relationships that came out of this experience continue to this day. In 1988, I helped organize and lead a disaster team from Seattle to the Soviet Republic of Armenia after an earthquake devastated that region. I was also medical director of the Goodwill Games in 1990 in Seattle and was able to facilitate a huge physicians' exchange between Soviet doctors and doctors in the western part of the state of Washington."

"From all of these trips to Russia I realized that, apart from our cultural differences, we are all pretty much the same human beings. What unites us is so much more than anything that separates us in terms of culture. I have dedicated a lot of my spare time attempting to do something about the insanity of a national defense policy of mutually assured destruction, when in one push of a button we could wipe out civilization. Many of my other activities have sprung from this commitment."

Roy finds that a balance of medicine and community involvement contributes to a sense of life purpose. His credentials and creditability as a physician are beneficial in going out into the community to discuss some of the broader issues.

"As chair of the Washington State Medical Association's violence prevention committee, I involve myself in issues relating to domestic violence and youth gun violence. We developed materials for physicians to give to women who come in for medical treatment resulting from physical abuse. When doctors ask the right questions and get a positive response, our materials provide the tools they need to help victims and expand their options. Often, the medical community is the only opportunity a woman may have to speak to someone if she has a very controlling spouse."

"If it is possible to deal with the stresses of medicine, I believe it must be done by restructuring our work around some other values."

—David Hilfiker, MD
Healing the Wounds (1985)

He also founded, with the Seattle police department, a program called *Cops and Docs*, that teaches junior high school students about the medical and legal consequences of using guns. They have educated more than 8,000 students over the past 5 years in the Seattle Public School District. The 2-day program uses actual pictures of gun violence cases from a trauma center to stimulate thinking among students about the real medical consequences of gun violence as compared with what they see on television, which is very unrealistic.

Roy Farrell's story reminds us of the Great Commandment, central to almost all religious traditions in one form or another, calling us to love God, neighbor, and self. In terms of vocation, Richard Bolles in his book, *What Color Is Your Parachute?*, states it in this manner:

> "[Part of our mission on earth]...is to exercise that Talent which you came to Earth to use in those place(s) or setting(s) which God has caused to appeal to you the most, and for those purposes which God most needs to have done in the world." [7]

Roy came into medicine through a back door. As a child, Roy suffered from asthma. "I would miss school 10 or 20 days a year because of asthmatic attacks. As a result of this, I saw doctors more often than I cared to. I went through a series of desensitization

---

[7] Bolles R. *What Color Is Your Parachute?* Berkeley, CA: Ten Speed Press; 2000: 368.

injections once a week for what seemed to be years. Therefore, I had more exposure to medicine than most people. I started out in college in electrical engineering and enlisted in the Navy ROTC. In the mid-60s I was headed to flying jet airplanes off of an aircraft carrier in the South China Sea had I remained in the ROTC. Somehow during my college education, I became interested in the life sciences and was much more attracted to biology and biochemistry than I was to engineering. I came to realize that I was much more of a people person and not interested in walking around campus with a slide rule. I could have satisfied my need to relate to people by moving into aviation or business, but I was simply fascinated by the medical sciences, how the body functions and how to diagnose and treat diseases. I actually graduated with a degree in electrical engineering, but managed to get a medical discharge from the Navy because of asthma and went to medical school. I was like Robert Frost's road less traveled. I jumped on a new path and never looked back."

"Where your talents and the needs of the world cross, there lies your vocation."

—Aristotle

We asked Roy about what led him into the emergency department as opposed to other specialties.

"I thought about that many times. I started out to be an orthopedic surgeon. I liked it, but during the first year of my residency, I discovered that what I really enjoyed the most was the emergency department. The only way I could describe it was 'exhilarating, challenging, and gratifying.' So, I decided to move in this direction. That was back when it was not identified as a formal specialty and before there were special training programs available. Many of us simply decided to work in the ER and we created our own training programs as it evolved. I ended up being the president of the state chapter of the American College of Emergency Physicians."

He adds, "It [emergency medicine] suits my personality very well. I am somewhat of a stimulus addict. I like the fact that I don't know what is coming in the door next and that each day is unique. I am challenged by what occurs because the scope of what I am confronted with is so broad. Even when there are common conditions such as appendicitis, I must be on my toes and use all of the skills I have in terms of practical knowledge and intuition to make sure I don't miss the unusual case. I actually enjoy it when things are just on the verge of being out of control.

I delight in responding to five things at once and determining which needs my attention first."

Roy believes that having the opportunity to take advantage of the sabbatical offered by the hospital where he practices has been very important to him as an emergency department physician.

"We have an opportunity to take a sabbatical leave after 10 years for 12 months at 30% of our salary. Our job is waiting for us when we come back as long as we can find someone acceptable to the department to fill in while we are gone. Every 7 years thereafter we can take another sabbatical. Not everyone takes advantage of this benefit or takes the entire 12 months, but just knowing that you have this option is a source of tremendous mental peace. It provides a sense of knowing that you are not trapped in your job. I have been in this one job for the past 24 years and, truthfully, I could not have done it without the opportunity to take leave occasionally to do other things."

"Some of the other things I have done include working for a year in an academic trauma center at the University of California, Irvine. I got to experience a different practice environment from my practice in Seattle, working on more knife and gunshot wounds. During that year I wrote a textbook in emergency medicine, which I could not have accomplished under ordinary circumstances."

"Another time, I took 4 months off. My wife and I home-schooled our 12-year-old son that year. I bought a motor home and we drove around the US, putting 15,000 miles on the vehicle. We visited almost all of the national parks in the country and many of the historical sites. We used this as an opportunity to educate our son about the geography and history of the US, as well as keeping him up on the other disciplines. It was a tremendous family experience."

Roy believes that sabbaticals are wonderful ways to help physicians maintain their passion for the profession and to avoid burnout. He also thinks that all medical schools should help their senior students, before they apply for their residencies, to get some idea about who they are through the use of the Myers-Briggs Type Indicator® and other career-assessment processes.

"We could offer some counseling about what specialties are good fits for them in medicine. You are not telling them what they can or cannot do, but giving them a better sense of how their personalities match with the various alternatives. Most of us sort of stumble into a specialty somewhat blindfolded. All we do now is throw people into 6-week clinical rotations in medical school and let them sort it out themselves."

At the time of our interview, Roy was 54 years old and had been practicing medicine for 27 years. He believes that he has grown over the years, especially in a spiritual sense. "I am more comfortable talking about a wider range of issues with my patients. For example, I am much more at ease talking to patients about the spiritual connotations of their illness and about end-of-life issues. I trust my intuition more today than in the past."

Along these lines, Roy believes a good physician obviously must be technically competent. "Especially for those of us who are generalists," he emphasizes, "it involves knowing when to ask for help."

Beyond this, he states that a good physician maintains awareness that it is a great privilege to serve patients in an inclusive manner, knowing also that there are alternative ways of healing. "A good doctor realizes that body, mind, and spirit interact. When relating to patients, I find it does not require a lot of extra time to be more inclusive in this respect."

We asked Roy about where he believes the power to heal resides. He said, "So many patients come into the emergency department in physical and/or emotional distress. The nurse will check them in and put the chart in the rack. The physician can pick up the chart, enter the room, and after about 5 or 10 minutes, the patient is usually much calmer. The physical examination is just a laying on of hands. I don't put myself out as someone who heals in this manner, but there is benefit to the therapeutic touch."

In *The Youngest Science, Notes of a Medical-Watcher,* Lewis Thomas, MD, concurs:

"There, I think, is the oldest and most effective act of doctors, the touching. Some people don't like being handled by others, but not, or almost never, sick people. They *need* being touched, and part of the dismay of being very sick is the lack of close human contact. Ordinary people, even close friends, even family members, tend to stay away from the very sick, touching them as infrequently as possible for fear of interfering, or catching the illness, or just fear of bad luck. The doctor's oldest skill in trade was to place his hands on the patient." [8]

[8] Thomas L. *The Youngest Science, Notes of a Medicine-Watcher.* New York, NY: Viking Press; 1983: 56.

Today, the practice of healing touch is gaining popularity because our highly developed medical technology requires the balance of human touch and intuitive perception. It involves a systematic approach to healing using energy interventions that incorporate a variety of therapeutic maneuvers such as massage. Now endorsed by American Holistic Nurses' Association and sponsored through Healing Touch International (HTI), the training offers a multilevel training experience that incorporates selected interventions to affect the human energy system.

Beyond touch, Roy says, "In the final analysis, the essence of healing is spiritual. In fact, there are studies showing that prayer does seem to make a positive difference. In particular, Dr Larry Dossey writes prolifically about controlled studies demonstrating prayer contributes to healing. In my work with patients one-on-one, I attempt to give them an opportunity to address their spiritual situation. Occasionally, a patient will ask me to pray for them and I do. It is important to convey to them that the doctor honors their sacred orientations. Clearly, there are many examples of the miraculous healing of cancer and other diseases that seem to disappear for no reason."

With respect to the current health care environment in general, Roy believes that our system is dysfunctional.

"If any intelligent group of citizens were given the task of designing a health care system for our country, they would never come up with something like what we have today. It is irrational, unfair, and, in many situations, unworkable. Given the amount of resources we put into it, it simply does not serve society very well. Politically, I am firmly convinced that things will have to get worse before they get better. At this time, we have 45 million people in this country who are uninsured. The next recession, and there will always be one, will likely increase this figure to 65 or 70 million people. Because of having a pre-existing condition, the people who do have insurance and who develop a medical problem are often afraid to quit their jobs because they will lose their insurance. Our freedom to make choices remains altered and limited in many instances by a jury-rigged system."

"The political will in Congress and in state legislatures doesn't exist to make the fundamental changes required. There are too many self-interest groups preventing structural reform. Therefore, short-term pessimism prevails on my part. At some point, the situation will deteriorate to the point that the American public will demand change in the way we finance and insure health care."

"In addition, it is disruptive and anxiety-producing at a minimum to force patients who have established a long-term trusting relationship with their physician to change because their employer chooses a different insurance. I provide my services under a staff model HMO where we have the full range of medical specialties. We are insulated from many of the frustrations that physicians in private practice experience with managed care. Our physicians do make the medical decisions without having to get prior authorization. We have an attitude of mutual cooperation in helping a patient receive the service needed. So, I personally do not get a lot of frustrated patients as might occur in other HMOs."

As we completed the interview, Roy again underlined the importance of maintaining a spiritual focus.

"If we don't have a spiritual focus, I think we experience a void of some kind. Without this [in any vocation], we are not really sure of why we are here or who we are as a person. As a doctor, it is very easy to be misled into perceiving oneself primarily as a privileged professional with a nice house in a nice area of the town, or something like that. Without a spiritual focus to anchor who you really are as a human being on this earth, you easily can be led astray."

Passionate Activist

Judith Eve Lipton, MD

Surrounded by floor-to-ceiling bookshelves and overlooking the yard and corral at their farm, it is not hard to imagine Dr Judy Lipton's interests.

"I just adore animals," she says by way of explanation. "I'm inescapably drawn to orphaned kittens or puppies. I have four horses, four dogs, three cats, and a turtle," she laughs. "I used to take in orphaned kittens and bottle-feed them."

Judy's decision to enter medical school in 1971 was more by default than design, she confesses. Nor, does she view her path into medicine and ultimately into psychiatry as being particularly romantic. "The truth is," she reports, "I got married at the age of 18 and gave birth to a child at 19 while I was a junior in college."

Very quickly it became evident that her marriage would fail and she would have no physical means of support. She majored in chemistry, and her parents were both physicians, so it seemed like the most natural thing in the world was to be a physician instead of a waitress.

"My good grades helped me to get into medical school," she says. "However, my baby posed a problem, but the dean of the school at the University of North Carolina, Chapel Hill, Dr Ike Taylor, supported me and believed in me even though I was a 19-year-old single parent taking care of a 1-year-old child."

Judy contemplated specializing in neonatology because she especially enjoyed watching babies being born. However, her very small hands limited her ability to conduct a pelvic examination. Also, her slight dyslexia would have made it difficult to be a surgeon.

"I rationalize my choice of psychiatry by saying I was more interested in people's love lives than in their livers," she declares. "And, it was true. I like to read a lot of novels and came to view psychiatry as comparable to reading 50 novels at one time, and even having a minor role to play in some of them. I like the stories and drama involved in my profession."

"But again," she confides, "there was a kind of default option involved in my choice. I wish my story were more romantic. In some ways, I might have been happier in something like internal medicine or pediatrics. However, my son was only 4 years old and I had completed 2 years of medical school being on call every other night or every third evening. I had horrific decisions to make about caring for my son and patients at the same time. I had to deal with baby-sitters getting sick or failing to show up. I remember one time during a surgical rotation when I was expecting to leave the hospital on a Saturday to pick up my son. One of my patients developed a GI bleed. The resident in charge asked me how I could possibly leave the hospital when my patient was experiencing problems. Yet, my son needed to be picked up from day care, so I was faced with an impossible dilemma. I had to call the day care and explain that I was going to be late again. It was a no-win situation. Sometimes I short changed my son and sometimes my patients. But I guess I made it through because I was a fast reader with a good memory."

"The on-call rotation in psychiatry was 1 in 7 nights. I chose it because I didn't perceive having the resources to do otherwise. I had to make a series of very practical choices," she admits.

In retrospect, apart from family challenges, Judy realizes that she experienced some personal abuse in medical school. "At the time," she says, "I didn't see the schedule as abusive, although I wish it had been different. Medical school was a boot camp. It involved many rites of initiation and a kind of purgatory. I know that I was sexually harassed several times, although I didn't know what it was about at the time. I took it for granted that this was how the world worked."

Although Judy was in private practice as a psychiatrist from 1980–1998, medicine has not been her passion. She admits, "I can't truthfully say I am passionate about medicine. I do know some of the things I am passionate about in the sense of a love affair." As previously mentioned, she is passionate about animals. "I hope my patients don't take offense at this, but I don't feel the same way about medicine. For me, it's more like housekeeping, a matter of doing something really important because it needs to be done. Doing medicine well makes me happy, but I feel a little grim about it. I come to medicine because it needs to be done and it's a noble profession."

Judy sometimes views passion in the sense of being in a fervent relationship, which is not always a wise relationship. Passion itself is not always a healthy thing; it can become an infatuation, a kind of mini-manic episode. She says, "People can do things that they are passionate about and can get into huge trouble. My older daughter is passionate about mountain climbing and I'm scared to death she will die prematurely in some accident or avalanche. She is inescapably drawn to the mountains; the higher, colder, and icier they are, the more she finds them intriguing. Where is the dividing line between passion and addiction? Passion can be different than a measured, intellectual choice."

She continues, "There exists another, higher level kind of passion. Some passionate decisions are not happy choices. For example, I am passionately committed to the prevention of nuclear war, but not because I like the topic. I hate the topic of nuclear war. I'm bored and tired with the subject. If all the world's nuclear weapons were suddenly dismantled and I didn't have to invest energy on the issue, I would be thrilled to pieces. I will continue to fight against nuclear war, but it is a grim kind of passion."

The more Judy talked of her intense passion against nuclear weapons, it appeared clear that the *element of involvement* is her passion. Smiling, she admits that she has an affinity for the Cowardly Lion in *The Wizard of Oz*. Although she does not seek out important issues to take on, she cannot *not* become involved when she sees a need and thinks that she can make a difference.

Her intense opposition to nuclear arms proliferation led her to respond to a 1979 ad in a Boston newspaper placed by the Physicians for Social Responsibility. The movement began in 1963 at Harvard because of atmospheric nuclear testing and was propelled by the Cuban missile crisis. In 1979, she was asked by Helen Caldicott, its founder and one of the country's most ardent nuclear activists, to start a chapter in Washington State. Judy went off the Washington Physicians for Social Responsibility board in the early 1990s but has recently returned for another term.

Today, Judy speaks of being spiral bound in her career. After practicing psychiatry for 18 years, she closed her practice. She found herself fatigued, and her husband was encouraging her to write more books with him. To date, they have written three books together, two of them about nuclear war.

Their first was *Stop Nuclear War, a Handbook* published in 1982 as a guide for antinuclear activists and nominated for an American Book Award. The second, *The Caveman and the Bomb*, released in 1984, dealt with the psychology of the arms race. Their third book, *Making Sense of Sex, Why Men and Women are Different*, became available in 1997. The latter two books focus on evolutionary biology.

Judy and her husband have been working together for 20 years in a field now being called evolutionary psychology. For 15 years they have been working on a fourth book titled *Passing the Pain Along*, which addresses the phenomenon of redirected aggression, looking at the behavior of both animals and humans. She explains this phenomenon with an example. "When one horse kicks another, the second horse will kick a third horse down on the pecking order. You can see this behavior played out in many different species and certainly with humans. Having a scapegoat is a way to stabilize stress hormones."

This book remains uncompleted because, she says, "I discover that I get lonely writing at home. Secondly, I developed a back pain disorder, so sitting hour after hour causes considerable pain. A third consideration is needing to earn more money."

At this time, Judy is in the process of reinventing her career. As we spoke, her direction was being fabricated. Her part-time practice currently involves geriatric psychiatry. Working with several different nursing homes, she meets with elderly residents, their families, and with the nursing staff. "My goal is to make the elderly as comfortable as possible as their days begin to wane," she says.

At the moment, her main career objective is focused on creating a position in a local hospital to develop a psychosocial support program for women with breast cancer. In addition, she hopes to develop a private practice in the evolving new field of psycho-oncology, applying psychiatry to cancer patients. "It's very cool," she explains, "Not all cancer patients need psychosocial support services. However, interesting literature suggests that, when people with martial problems, stress, or depression are treated, there is some evidence that cancer will not reoccur or will be less severe. I'm excited, and if it goes well, instead of having a job as a psychiatrist in a private office, which can be rather intense and lonely at times, I may be in a more communal setting. I would see patients in medical exam rooms, as well as when they are receiving chemotherapy treatments or waiting for radiation. Some I may see in the hospital when they are sick or in hospice when they are dying. In any case, I'll be moving around and will be part of a team."

"And, the really cool thing is that I'm writing a grant proposal to actually do group therapy for couples, where the wife has breast cancer. It turns out that many couples break up because of body image problems and weight gain or loss when one person develops breast cancer. There can also be a negative relation between having a mastectomy and one's sexual activity. Many women lose both their breasts and their husbands, along with financial security. I hope to help people communicate and deal emotionally with such problems, especially with underserved women and their families who are without insurance. I am thrilled and passionate about it because it seems like it would be so helpful to people."

We asked Judy how she came to enter this new career path, whether she had received any professional guidance. "Not really! I've talked to a lot of people and have done extensive networking. Actually, this program came about because a friend who is a breast surgeon suggested that I speak with the director of the oncology program. Dreams begin to crystallize when you get a group of people to speak about possibilities," she declares.

In addition to and as part of her practice, Judy has worked with other physicians who were distressed. She has provided consultations for the Physicians Health Program in Washington State.

"In fact," Judy says, "Lynn Hankes (whose story is included in this book) and I will be offering a program shortly. I will speak about sex differences and he will speak about fragile physicians. It's fun to put together new programs and new ideas. Physician wellness is one of my passions!"

Judy believes that physicians need all the help they can get right now. Sadly, she says, "A lot of physicians entered medicine with a passionate commitment and vision of being the next Albert Schweitzer. Today they have been ground down and chewed up by a mismanaged health care system. They are fairly depressed because of the vocational passion seeping out of their lives. They entered the profession rather idealistically, but now often find themselves in an assembly line, 'doc-in-a-box' environment. Often, they don't know where to turn to get help. It's humiliating. On top of this, it used to be that when it came time to have your license renewed, if you checked a box indicating that you had seen a counselor or received mental health services, it could hold up the relicensing process. Only recently has this little check box been removed from the application. But even today, doctors are asked intrusive questions for licensure. So, getting help in this current health care system is not very easy. Also, there is a lot of denial in the medical community. I have a friend who lectures on physician burnout. As director of psychiatry at a local hospital, he attempted to offer support groups for doctors, but no one wants to come."

During the course of treating serious illness, physicians must also deal with personal trauma. Judy underscores that many physicians observe horrific events and pain with some of their patients. She reports that survivor syndromes develop with physicians, something similar to battle fatigue, because they witness things like car accidents, child abuse, or backyard abortions. Losing a patient may result in personal trauma, especially if a physician has cared for that person over a period of time.

Changing the subject to the process of healing, Judy shares how she would define this complex issue. She believes that physical healing can occur at several levels. For example, a wound may heal itself with or without scar tissue. The same holds true for a psychological injury of some kind. Functionality can be restored, but often a scar remains, some evidence that the regeneration is imperfect.

As an atheist, Judy does not connect spirit and prayer with healing, although she knows that people in her practice do engage in prayer and religious practices. She would do nothing to encourage or discourage them and admits that for many, spirituality and prayer represent ways of coming to peace with what is happening to them. Judy notes that Tibetan chants, for example, are a form of self-soothing.

From her early career decision to her antinuclear activism and now to a reinvented and reenergized career, Judy's experiences reflect great determination and, though perhaps reluctantly, the courage to respond to need. As noted earlier, her passion, no matter the arena, revolves around being actively involved.

As we concluded our discussion, with some tears and a voice full of emotion, Judy shared one of the final paragraphs from *The Plague*, by Albert Camus. It speaks deeply to her and in many ways is at the core of who she is. It is as follows:

> Nonetheless, he knew that the tale he had to tell could not be one of a final victory. It could be only the record of what had to be done, and what assuredly would have to be done again in the never ending fight against terror and its relentless onslaughts, despite their personal afflictions, but all who, while unable to be saints but refusing to bow down to pestilences, strive their utmost to be healers. [9]

---

[9] Camus A. *The Plague*. Gilbert S, trans. New York, NY: Vintage Books; 1972: 287.

Innovative Educator and Wellness Doctor

Peter Ways, MD

Dr Peter Ways' enthusiasm as a young student entering Columbia University's School of Medicine in 1949 soon waned. He remembers finding the first 2 years an exercise in rote memory. He and his classmates were treated as objects, their humanity ignored by a faculty steeped in a herd mentality. Lecture halls were large and most of the instruction was boring. With rare exceptions, the information provided by teachers seemingly had little to do with the actual practice of medicine. On a few Saturday mornings, a clinician met with the students and presented a patient who demonstrated the connection between the classroom and the practice of medicine. But for the most part, as stated by Dr Larry Weed, a prominent medical educator, Peter and his fellow students were required to "learn all the answers before they knew what the questions were." They were expected to put in exhausting hours memorizing information only to regurgitate it during exams.

Exposed to their first cadavers, students mutilated bodies without any preparation or warning as to how this experience might impact their emotions and psyche. Gallows humor, unscheduled mutilations, and diminished or inappropriate emotional responsiveness were the result. These first 2 years awakened Peter's interest in the basic dilemmas of medical education.

However, opportunities did emerge that engaged his passion. For example, during the summer between his second and third year, Peter took an elective in the thyroid clinic at Massachusetts General Hospital with Ben Wright, a classmate. They also conducted animal research on thyroid physiology. This renewed an interest in research, a passion that would continue throughout his career.

Pediatrics was Peter's first clinical clerkship. "Two classmates and I showed up at 7:30 am the first day and were each immediately assigned four patients. I was led to Ned's crib by a nurse who said, 'Ned is 5 and has widespread neuroblastoma, a multicentric neurological tumor. He is not an easy patient to be with or take care of.' Despite her warning, I was totally unprepared for the grotesque lad I met. He was a miniature Quasimodo—the Hunchback of Notre Dame. Several orange- to grapefruit-sized tumor masses stuck out of his head, back, and abdomen."[10] Peter wasn't taught how to deal with the powerful and frightening emotions associated with such experiences.

After medical school, Peter moved to Seattle and began his internship and residency at Harborview Medical Center, then the only clinical site for the University of Washington Medical School. It was an intense learning experience and an incredibly difficult period of working many long hours. Even more than in medical school, he was presented with one situation after another that powerfully affected him emotionally and spiritually.

During his third month in internship, he treated a 78-year-old man in severe congestive heart failure. The man responded well to treatment and within a week was ready to be discharged. Peter had become quite fond of Joe and his wife. The day before Joe was to go home, Peter heard a bellow from the men's restroom. Joe had collapsed in one of the stalls and the only way to reach him was to climb over the top of the door. He suffered an acute heart attack and within an hour he was dead. Devastated and angry, Peter ran down the hall. "Sobbing fiercely, I told the head nurse I will never again get that close to a patient."

In the face of repeated heart-rending experiences, Peter began to bury his emotions and anesthetize his pain with alcohol and drugs, without support or a way to ventilate. "The environment blunted my physician spirit, so I succumbed to the spirits of alcohol."

The 6 years of medical school internship and residency, when he was engaged primarily in treating patients, continued to be profoundly stressful, demoralizing, and lonely. "I loved taking care of people, relating to them, and watching them get better, but my passion was gradually eroded by the pain, isolation, and lack of emotional and spiritual support." Peter and two of his colleagues have since published a book titled *Clinical Clerkships: The Heart of Professional Development* that speaks to these issues in some detail. [11]

Reflecting on a different subject, Peter speaks about seeking to connect with his "true self" throughout his career rather than his "should self." Jim uses similar terminology when working with clients in career counseling.

---

[10] Ways P, Engel J, Finkelstein P. *Clinical Clerkships: The Heart of Professional Development*. Thousand Oaks, CA: Sage Publications, Inc; 2000: 12–13.
[11] Ways P, Engel J, Finkelstein P. *Clinical Clerkships: The Heart of Professional Development*. Thousand Oaks, CA: Sage Publications, Inc; 2000.

The *should self* generally responds to external messages about life and how it should be lived. It contains messages we received from parents and other significant adults who influenced us during childhood, from peers who may have pigeonholed us through stereotyping, and from teachers who may have influenced us with their sometimes narrow or false assumptions.

The *should self* often contains what Michael Ray calls the "Voice of Judgment (VOJ)" that expresses itself through self talk or in harsh communication with others.[12] Peter and his colleagues report the following scenario in their book, a sad example of the VOJ in medicine (one of them actually witnessed this):

> A man was admitted with a new myocardial infraction (MI). The resident arrived at the bedside to insert a central venous pressure line. Still in some pain, the patient was restless and moved his arm as the procedure was beginning.
>
> "Hold still, you ___hole," said the resident.
>
> The patient had a cardiac arrest. Cardiopulmonary resuscitation was unsuccessful. He died! [13]

On the other hand, the *true self* serves as an internal messenger of wisdom and stimulates our compassion and creative energies. Expressions of this inner wisdom can be found in almost all cultures. Some Native American Indians called it the Familiar Voice. In Eastern religions, it could be Zen Buddhism's Original Face and in Christian traditions, the Christ Self. The psychologist Carl Jung named this inner messenger his Million Year Old Man.

Attempting to be true to himself and others, Peter has had difficulty conforming to external standards. Generally, old paradigms do not work for him and he seeks new paradigms, which is part of his maverick makeup. During his internship, Peter became uncommonly interested (for an intern) in how to prevent disease as opposed to curing it. He also became more and more interested in the process of medical education and its shortcomings. For this reason, he left Seattle for Michigan State University's College of Human Medicine to pursue opportunities as a medical educator.

---

[12] Ray M, Myers R. *Creativity in Business.* New York, NY: Doubleday; 1989.

[13] Ways P, Engel J, Finkelstein P. *Clinical Clerkships: The Heart of Professional Development.* Thousand Oaks, CA: Sage Publications, Inc.; 2000: 63.

Many educators act on the assumption that knowledge is transmitted to people. A common image depicts information pouring into someone's head. However, the term "to educate" literally means "to bring forth." Therefore, some believe education involves bringing forth the knowledge in someone that already unconsciously exists in him or her and in the universe (ie, bringing it into consciousness). In Peter's words, the best education is "learning by discovery, which is more effective and more human. I love this approach to education."

In *Clinical Clerkships*, Peter and his colleagues relate how intellectual vitality is often squashed during medical school. "Its salient characteristics are curiosity, creativity, the capability for divergent thinking, integrative capacity, and tolerance for ambiguity." [14]

Andrew Hunt, MD, former dean of Michigan State University's medical school, serves as one of Peter's heroes. Says Peter, "Dr Hunt is extremely honest. He admits when he doesn't know something. Most of all, he gave me and other faculty members both permission and the resources needed to be creative. This was a kind of trust that I had never encountered in an administrative educator before."

> "I tried to learn everything and I just couldn't. Now I try to figure out what they're going to test me on and learn that...it's a bitter pill; it goes against my values to study for grades."
>
> —Second year student
> Clinical Clerkships (2000)

With Andy's support and guidance, Peter conceived and implemented Focal Problems, "the first major commitment to early, integrated, problem-based learning in any medical school." This approach to education contrasts sharply with the traditional curriculum that requires thousands of pieces of information in preparation for exams.

Alfred North Whitehead also stands tall in Peter's mind. "*The Aims of Education and Other Essays* is a great book, first published in 1929. It makes so much sense," notes Peter. "Whitehead defines education as the acquisition of the art of the utilization of knowledge." Whitehead states, "There is only one subject-matter for education, and that is Life in all its manifestations...students are alive, and the purpose of education is to stimulate and guide their self-development." [15]

---

[14] Ways P, Engel J, Finkelstein P. *Clinical Clerkships: The Heart of Professional Development.* Thousand Oaks, CA: Sage Publications, Inc; 2000: 141.
[15] Whitehead AN. *The Aims of Education and Other Essays.* New York, NY: Macmillan; 1929: 10.

Peter emphasizes that such statements are completely congruent with his personal educational philosophy. "Learning how to
use information and use it well is what education is all about, not
simply the memorization of material," he affirms. "This opens the
door for spirit and soul to enter into teaching and learning. It also
implies that the teacher is more of a facilitator than an authoritative source of expertise. It doesn't mean to imply that the teacher
is unimportant, but that the teacher is not all-important."

Recently, Peter, with Lura Pethlel and John Engel, facilitated
a course on spirituality and medicine at Northeastern Ohio
University's College of Medicine. Using their creative skills, facilitating this course for medical students has been an unusually
innovative and soulful experience for the "instructor." The
process is a concrete example of learning through discovery.
Peter and his faculty colleagues enjoyed this so much that they
concluded, "it doesn't seem like work."

Peter and his teaching partner Lura Pethlel begin by using a
questionnaire to explore student perceptions about spirituality.
One question elicits the differences between spirituality and religion. Another gathers information about the characteristics of
people viewed by the student as being spiritual. Still a third
question addresses the similarities and differences between spirit
and soul. Then, during the sessions, students are asked to give
short presentations on their personal "model" of spirituality. Use
of icons, pictures, and various other "props" is encouraged but
cannot be intellectualized. For example, one student described
how her spiritual development is like the making of a quilt.
Another constructed an origami. Questions from the other class
members are welcome, but must be asked for clarification only;
they cannot be adversarial. Thereafter, the medical students conduct interviews with "programmed patients" who have been
recruited for this purpose and who may or may not have an
actual medical problem.

This technique is used more and more in medical education,
although in this course, the interview is spiritually oriented.
With major input from the class, a composite approach is syn-
thesized to determine when and how best to explore spiritual
issues with patients.

"The whole thrust of this course was to give medical students
as beginning clinicians permission and encouragement to explore
the spiritual dimension whenever it seemed appropriate," says

Peter. "The other objective is to give students some practice with the tools of initiating such conversations."

Like many of us, Peter struggles with attempting to arrive at an explicit definition of spirit and soul. Peter does associate the words with some kind of linkage. "For me, spirituality means connection and communication, whether through prayer, meditation, or other mediums. Soul helps me connect with deeper parts of myself and to the external world."

In his 70s, Peter resists the concept of retirement. He will continue to focus upon the spiritual dimension of medicine and upon helping doctors to take care of themselves. He is currently unsure of how this will play itself out and is involved in a path of discernment. He speaks of Parker Palmer and how he waited for the right door to open in his life.[16] Palmer went to a wise woman in a Quaker community with the frustration that he had been searching for vocational direction for more than 2 years and nothing had appeared. The woman replied that she was 62 years old and nothing had opened for her either, but that a lot of doors had closed behind her and this was valuable.

Wherever Peter's continuing journey takes him, we suspect that he will be engaged in innovative education. We also imagine it will involve facilitating "high touch" among human beings.

---

[16] Palmer PJ. *Let Your Life Speak; Listening for the Voice of Vocation.* San Francisco, CA: Jossey-Bass; 1999.

Change Agent

Jean H. Marshall, MD

Dr Jean Marshall views one of the benefits of being in family practice as providing a continuity of care for more than one generation. Although she does not deliver babies, she has seen many children grow up during her 19 years in family practice.

"One of my patients whom I began seeing at age 7 or 8 now has children of her own," Jean recounts with a smile. "Family doctors really do well at providing this kind of continuity of care. It is a matter of managing, preventing, coordinating, and optimizing health over a life span. Of course, I see many more women than men, probably because I am one of them. I also allow my patients to talk. I believe they know they are listened to and can discuss issues more comfortably with a woman." She adds with a laugh, "This is also why I am always behind in my schedule."

In our earlier book, *Reclaiming Soul in Health Care*, we discussed two worldviews. The first is that the universe operates like a clock or a machine. The second is based on theoretical physics, suggesting that the universe is more like a living web. We asked Jean to comment on these views and to share her perspectives.

Responding thoughtfully, she says, "I lean toward the latter viewpoint in the sense that one change impacts others. I find myself always speaking about and appreciating the many life dynamics affecting people's health. Much of it is unrelated to bacteria or the physical environment, but has more to do with an individual's physical behavior and mental–emotional processes. It impacts other risk factors to one's health. The issue is, what predisposes one to illness, creating a scenario that leads to a disease or an accident? So, in this sense everything is interconnected and you can't simply look at a person in isolation. Of course, I'm not in a position time-wise to explore all of the factors affecting a person's health, but I do have an appreciation of the interplay of factors."

She continues, "What I like to do with my patients involves feeding back to them the reality of this interplay of factors. They have at least some control over these dynamics. People often have more control over their lives than they might think. For example, driving a car represents the greatest risk factor for patients between the ages of early teen years up through age 45. A person has at least some control over when, where, and how to drive an automobile. In addition, a lot of an individual's anger and depression stems from feeling loss of control. Most of us have more control over life than we are willing to accept."

"The one thing I bring to my patients is the knowledge and skills needed to become more assertive and positive in their approach to life as opposed to being negative. I participated in an Outward Bound event when I was 16 years old, learning how to overcome mental obstacles. I learned that if you really want to do something, you'd find a way to do it. I question people who make excuses for why their lives are miserable, or why they are unhappy. I want them to realize that they can do so much more than they think they can do."

"You don't have choices unless you have at least three."

—Jane Clarke
Stress Management
Counselor
Dallas, Texas

Reflecting on her perception of soul and its relationship to spirituality, Jean explains, "I view these words as not relating solely to religious issues. Without a doubt, there exist other energies outside the purely physical, biological, and scientific dimensions of life. I *do not* believe that if you can't measure it, it's not real. Of course, we have almost limitless ways to measure and dissect phenomena to establish principles and laws for perceived reality. However, there remains an additional component beyond what can be measured, the spiritual dimension."

Jean believes that soul relates more to people than to things. "In some ways soul could be the inner, mental, and emotional makeup of a person. It remains beyond our understanding. A person's individuality and values reflect his or her soul."

As we have heard during interviews with other physicians, and perhaps without giving considerable thought to it, Jean intuitively captures one of the premier characteristics of soul as we understand it. In part, soul describes the essence of who we are as unique individuals. No two persons or "souls" are alike. Or, if you like, we are all abnormal in some sense. In *Boundaries of the Soul*, June Singer says, "To be 'normal' means the same as being able and willing to conform to some sort of socially produced 'norm,' an 'accepted' standard of behavior."[17]

---

[17] Singer J. *Boundaries of the Soul*. New York, NY: Anchor Books; 1973: 14.

The early experiences leading Jean into medicine were not particularly dramatic. There were no personal or family illnesses, nor did a mentoring adult steer her in this direction. She did very well in her study of the sciences, seeming to have an innate aptitude for them and was rewarded for performing well. She planned to enter a field of scientific research. But, she realized after a year of graduate study and sitting in a laboratory all alone much of the time that there was something missing in her career choice.

Warmly, she relates, "I missed interacting with people. Also, in order to be involved in basic research, I would have to live in a fairly large urban area. At that time, I thoroughly enjoyed backpacking and mountain climbing. Travel also intrigued me. I wanted to be able to go any place in the world and know that my set of skills would be valued. Therefore, I decided to enter medicine."

Paradoxically, she entered a staff model health maintenance organization (HMO) practice in an urban area right out of residency, so she hasn't actualized her entire dream. Meeting and marrying her husband impacted the decision. Had she been single, she might have pursued a contract in Nepal to provide medical assistance. But, she doesn't regret the decision. Just after we interviewed her, Jean departed on a 100-day round-the-world voyage with her daughter and other students who will receive college credits for the education gained from visiting many different countries. Jean was the physician for the ship.

At the time of her medical training, Jean found some of the older male physicians remaining tied to the belief that a woman's place is in the home. Also, when she got to the wards, she was expected to assume the role of mother to the patients. "Being in control, portraying analytical authoritative behaviors were viewed as unfeminine," she reports. "I wrote it off to an expression of society as a whole at the time. This view of having such differences between men and women was just beginning to significantly recede. In reality, I received a lot of encouragement for pursuing medicine. Brought about because of a lawsuit, 33% of us were women in my medical class, jumping from a previous high of 18%."

She continues, "I also found medical school rather easy. I was a lot more mature when I entered it. I had completed a year of postgraduate work, honing my learning skills and engaging in some traveling, so I was ready for the experience. Since I did well, perhaps I wasn't confronted with some of the stress felt by other students."

Interestingly, Jean found during her training that the nursing
staff at the hospital did not respond to her as favorably as to men.
Nurses sometimes viewed being asked to do something as being
unreasonable or authoritarian. Two factors probably surfaced
from these experiences.

"First, women expect women to communicate differently than
men," she believes. "With women, it is more of a collaborative
relationship, as in 'we're working together.' A man's mode of
communication is more hierarchical; 'I'll tell you what to do.' So
when a woman listens to another woman speaking, she is more
prepared to listen, expecting the two of them to work together."

"As a physician, sometimes I am more direct," she confesses,
"using a male tone and saying, 'I need this done right now.' Then
I get resistance from the nurses, as if I were somehow putting
them down as inferior. Of course, I don't mean to do this, but
I tend to be very direct. When I want to say something, I'll say it.
However, sometimes women aren't used to this kind of behavior
from other women. This serves as a kind of classic problem and
it's something we have to work on together, female physician and
staff alike. On my part, I work to use more inclusive language,
such as 'we've got this patient with a problem, so let's work
together on helping him. What are your ideas?'"

Jean's comments led us to reflect on masculine and feminine
archetypes. A word coined by C.G. Jung, *archetypes* are powerful
images and energies residing in all people. Masculine and feminine energies are way up in the hierarchy of such powers, existing to a greater or lesser degree in both women and men.
Feminine energies are more relationship oriented and masculine
energies more directive. In people like Jean, whom we perceive to
be quite advanced in terms of her psychological development,
one finds these energies more integrated and balanced. She can be
compassionate *and* directive. Similarly, with many of the male
physicians whom we interviewed, we find the feminine energies
emerging and incorporated with masculine energies.

Over the years, Jean feels she has grown and changed in terms
of practicing medicine. She explains, "I've had to change because
patients have far different expectations today than in earlier
times. More interaction is expected of doctors. Patients want more
information and more shared decision making."

Also, Jean believes that patients are developing much more of
an adversarial position; patients versus physicians. "More and

more, doctors are becoming identified with the health care system in general and specifically with the insurance system," she claims. "In terms of health insurance, perhaps initially we didn't think it would be bad because we thought we would be helping the patient make the best decision within the context of their coverage, but patients are much more demanding. They are encouraged to question our counsel."

Such an atmosphere caused Jean to develop new skills and tools in her practice to meet her patients' need for information and to increase participation in medical decision making.

"Family physicians always have been a bit less authoritative," Jean observes. "So, perhaps we have less change to go through than other specialties. The posture of blind faith used to make it more possible to be the knowledgeable expert."

Being in a staff model HMO, Jean feels she experiences a different kind of change with respect to managed care. "Being a family physician in a managed care environment offers almost an optimal situation. Managed care really supports our goal, which is to keep patients healthy. All of the factors in terms of how I make decisions are aligned around this," she declares.

"We help to keep people healthy within the context of knowing there is a limited pot of money available. Sometimes patients challenge us, suggesting we are simply attempting to save financial resources. But, why spend the money on a treatment that won't make any positive difference? If we did, we couldn't use the funds for something else. So we optimize patients' health within the context of limited resources."

Jean sees her role as one that connects individual patient care to the community's health as a whole, the use of antibiotics serving as an example.

"The more antibiotics we prescribe, the more likely resistant bacteria will surface. The more the resistant bacteria, the more the overall community suffers. Immunization is a classic example as well," she says expanding her thesis. "It may be low risk for you to get the shot, but if you get the shot, it lowers the level of disease and the costs to the whole community. Again, there is a limited pot of dollars. If we spend it all on one patient or all on one intervention, we aren't going to have money for other needs."

Jean considers herself equally optimistic and pessimistic about the future of health care. "I am optimistic," she asserts, "because we have better tools for making people healthier."

On the other hand, alluding to earlier concerns, she adds, "I am pessimistic because of the limited amount of money and the abuse of resources by many people. It's the selfish focus of what's in it for me. The external market-driven approach to medicine is going to create more have-nots and less-haves."

Jean readily confesses that medicine is not necessarily her passion. "My true passion is doing something that leads to positive change. I want to have a positive effect on the human race, and obviously to my patients, to my organization, and to my community. I am a person who likes to fix things, to come up with solutions that help people. Medicine is obviously a great area to be in if you like doing those things. However, there are other things I am more passionate about."

Pushed to identify her real passion, Jean laughs and answers, "I am more passionate about social causes. And, I can be passionate about activities rejuvenating my energy. A lot of that is gardening and cooking," she confesses. "I am tired after a day of medicine. I may be physically tired after gardening as well, but emotionally, I feel great afterward." She further explains passion as doing a greater good. She chuckles, "Maybe that's it; my passion has to be devoid of economics."

Like Roy Farrell, Jean has been involved in a community program called *Cops and Docs*. She explains, "About 8 years ago, I heard pediatrician Dr Fred Rivera present a paper that he co-authored that measured the deaths from guns in King County, Washington. They looked at the risk of death from firearm injuries, coming to the conclusion that for every firearm death involved in self-protection, there were two deaths caused by accidental injuries. People defending themselves with a gun were twice as likely to injure or kill themselves with their own gun. Forty-three percent of the time you were more likely to kill yourself, a family member, or friend than an unknown intruder with your own gun. It struck me that I didn't think most people knew that. It motivated me to become involved."

"When you try to tell adults about guns, they turn their intellects off and switch to their emotional, 'you are taking away a right' mode. But, kids are a great audience. Adults may change their behavior if it affects their kids."

Jean's involvement grew from working with the Washington Academy of Family Practitioners and from collaborating with Roy Farrell's work with the Seattle Police Department. The highly successful middle school program is beginning to spread to other areas and additional physicians are becoming involved.

Even though not a primary passion, medicine is obviously important to her. We wondered what Jean would do if she couldn't continue practicing.

"I'm sure it would be difficult," she acknowledges. "I would grieve and have a lot of anger. I would be challenged to take the knowledge and experience I have and use it in other ways, maybe not in direct patient care, but I would think how to use it. Maybe I would go into research, informing other doctors about what makes a difference in changing people's health. I have enough existing irons in the fire."

We commented that it would be easy for her to shift and use her skills in another capacity. She agreed, and then said softly, "But there would be grief and sadness."

WOUNDED HEALERS

"All strong souls first go to hell before they do the healing of the world they came here for. If we are lucky, we return to help those still trapped below."
—**Clarissa Estes**

The Naked Doctor

Bob Barnes, MD

In the opening chapter of his forthcoming book, tentatively titled *The Good Doctor is Naked*, Dr Bob Barnes describes in vivid detail a normal day in the life of a 10-year-old that turned out to be anything but normal. He left school one afternoon, skipping down the street, laughing, kidding, and playing with his buddies. Arriving home, he found that the street in front of his house, which on an ordinary day would have few cars, was lined with cars, bumper to bumper. He soon learned that the stock market had crashed and his father committed suicide. This tragic event would later lead to a journey toward grounding and transformation.

During his deep bout with depression, Parker Palmer, in his book, *Let Your Life Speak*, describes the way to God as being down. "I had always imagined God to be in the same general direction as everything else I valued: up [as in upbeat or uptown]. I had failed to appreciate the meaning of some words that had intrigued me since I first heard them in seminary—Tillich's description of God as the 'ground of being.' I had to be forced underground before I could understand that the way to God is not up but down." [1]

Bob wishes that he had begun his journey toward becoming grounded earlier in his career. Now retired after more than 30 years of practicing internal medicine, we asked him what he would do differently if he could start all over. Without hesitation, he says, "I would be trained in psychology and in spiritual formation in addition to the practice of medicine. I like to use the word 'grounded.' I would ground myself in who I am. I would hope that in medical school I would learn to accept myself in terms of my role and my limitations, and to avoid wearing a mask of power and perfectionism. This is why I'm calling my book, *The Good Doctor is Naked*. Even being like Uncle Joe could be a mistake; I would rather be myself."

After his father's death, his mother shipped Bob off to live with his uncle, who was a physician, in North Carolina. He recalls his uncle lovingly. "Uncle Joe was a big, stocky, red-haired man and

---

[1] Palmer P. *Let Your Life Speak, Listening for the Voice of Vocation.* San Francisco, CA: Jossey-Bass; 1999: 69.

the only doctor in a little town. He became my surrogate father and he loved me. I soon became the apple of his eye and he would brag about me in front of the people in the town. He took me by the hand and often let me join him during some of his home visits."

Memories of his uncle are rich with stories and lessons that made an impact on him as a small boy. "Traveling through country laced with cotton fields, to this day, I can visualize him taking the dog, Spot, and me in his Model-T Ford to see a patient," he says relating one such story.

"Now I become myself.
It's taken
Time, many years and places;
I have been dissolved and shaken,
Worn of other people's faces..."
—May Sarton
Now I Become Myself (1973)

"We went down a long dirt road to a shack with broken windows covered with newspapers. My uncle had delivered three other children for this Indian family. He was making a call to see the fourth baby he had recently delivered. He took me with him into the shack where the baby lay with a bandage wrapped around his stomach. There was a big lump inside the wrapping. Uncle Joe unwrapped the bandage, exposing a dead baby turtle on the navel of the baby. He told me later that some babies are born with jaundice and he had relented to the family's superstition that a turtle would correct the problem. I learned that day not to ignore such superstitions but to practice good medicine as well."

"I particularly remember the smells associated with Uncle Joe," he recalls fondly. "He smelled of iodine, chloroform, and ether. He was, and still is, my hero. Vocationally, there wasn't any question about it. I wanted to be like Uncle Joe. I didn't know that you had to look down a microscope or study chemistry to become a doctor. I just wanted to smell like him and carry a black bag." Not a little wistfully, Bob remembers that by the time he became a physician, those smells were gone.

In his early 80s, today Bob enjoys diversity in his life: Medicine, spirituality, writing, art, golf, tennis, travel, counseling individuals, public relations, teaching, and politics. This diversity and his expanded self-awareness were accelerated by a midlife crisis and a period of depression that happened when he was in his 50s.

"It began when I switched from practicing internal medicine to becoming director of medical education in a hospital. I introduced a quality care program that was rejected by most of the physicians. Belonging to a community is important to me, but I was often rejected by my peers. We all like to be accepted; it's important to one's self-image. It was very difficult for me to discover that when I spoke to a group of doctors about measuring the quality of their work, often a doctor would ask why I didn't back to practicing medicine again. That was hard on me and unexpected."

His disappointment soon turned into depression. "I didn't know how to handle my depression, but fortunately began to seek out assistance through therapy. I also visited with a priest who, like Uncle Joe, was also a kind of surrogate father to me. We talked about my experience a great deal. I had long talks with this priest and revisited childhood issues that developed with the loss of my father. Like other people, many doctors come from dysfunctional families and have histories of suffering because of it. Doctors do suffer, but they don't often have the time or energy to deal with it. I was lucky in having several mentors in this respect."

Bob's interest in spirituality and religion spans many years. "I had worked with the American Medical Association back in the 1960s on the topic of medicine and religion and had given talks to hospital groups, not about physicians' spirituality but about patient needs. That was also very difficult," Bob remembers,

"True art is never the offspring of formula, prescription or recipe, but the spontaneous expression of vital and individual feeling. The creative spirit can neither be legislated nor predicted. In the practice of medicine we must consciously separate the art from basic science and skills. A patient care review program must never destroy spontaneity, individuality, inventiveness or dissatisfaction with the status quo. . . . I see, through PCA [Patient Care Appraisal], the combined wisdom of many physicians being brought to bear on the needs of patients, while the one-to-one physician-patient relationship is respected and strengthened."

—Robert H. Barnes, MD
(Written as Director of the Health Care Review Center and reprinted with permission.)

"because doctors didn't want to get involved in such issues. But, I found out that it was very important to ask patients about their spirituality. It also quickly turned around with patients asking me about my experiences. Patients don't usually ask a doctor about his or her spiritual self, but physicians need to address this topic and often need help in learning how to approach it."

In retrospect, Bob thinks that shifting into the role of medical director where he experienced rejection might have been the best thing that ever happened. "Subsequently, I took a course in clinical pastoral education, and to my knowledge, I am still the only doctor, at least in the Northwest, who has done that. I learned about myself. My wife said that I became a better husband. My interest expanded significantly with the spiritual side of life. As part of my training, I was assigned to the AIDS ward. I visited with many patients who did not know, and I could not reveal to them, that I was a doctor, nor could I read the chart. It was very hard for me not to reveal that side of me," he confesses. "I wanted a tag on my lapel saying Robert H. Barnes, MD, Chief of Staff. All my tag said was 'Bob Barnes, Pastoral Care.' The other doctors couldn't imagine what I was doing. I was embarrassed to put the tag on."

It was also during this period of time when he stopped practicing medicine for a while and pursued other areas of interest. "I was so involved in quality of care that I became a candidate for the assistant secretary of health in Washington, DC. I was interviewed in the White House. In retrospect, I'm glad I didn't get the position. It settled some things for me, for example, the abortion issue. This was a time when Ronald Reagan was president and I didn't pass the litmus test. The second reason I didn't get the job was that I had never raised a million dollars for him," he says laughing.

"Actually, I was very passionate about working at a national level and I did so for 4 years as chairman of the National Committee on Vital and Health Statistics, which sounds like something boring. However, it turned into a wonderful experience because I learned about the importance of data in health care and its relationship to health policy. This group was an advisory committee to the secretary of health."

Cautioning against stereotyping five or six hundred thousand physicians, he describes qualities he believes make a good physician. "Of course, he or she always must be up-to-date in terms of his or her clinical practice, which is difficult to do in this day and age. The worst thing would be to enlist the services of a friendly doctor who doesn't know anything."

"Beyond technical competence, a good doctor knows himself and knows his role and his gifts. He or she is able to communicate and to ask for help when it is needed. The essential thing is to become aware of oneself as a human being who just happens to be a physician. He or she must be mature enough to take off one's mask of authority and power and infallibility.

"Related to that, you must face up to one's own humanity with a sense of humility. It involves the heart and soul." Regretfully, he continues, "I didn't learn this until later in my life. I was pushed hard to keep up with the business of medicine and the challenge to be a good clinician."

Virtually all of the physicians we interviewed for this book concur about the importance of listening. Bob says research indicates that the average physician interrupts a patient every 20 seconds. "We may not even be aware of it and, of course, there is some reason for it, because we are attempting to get enough information to solve a problem. However, this can actually get in the way of listening. Sometimes doctors have their own agendas and may jump to an early and sometime inaccurate conclusion. Or there may be multiple problems involved in a patient's situation that are not discovered. It is quite a skill to keep an open mind and let a patient speak until he is through talking. Sometimes a doctor will decide what he wants to say even before entering the room. Today I feel sorry that many doctors are so busy, but this is a necessity in the practice of medicine."

"'Dr Levine said that I have TS.'
'Yes, of course you have TS,'
*   I [Dr Lown] affirmed.*
She began to cry quietly.
'What do you think TS means?'
*   I inquired.*
'It means terminal situation.'
I told her that TS was an
*   abbreviation for tricuspid*
*   stenosis, but she was no*
*   longer listening.'"*

—Bernard Lown, MD
The Lost Art of Healing (1996)

Bob feels so strongly about the importance of listening that he would revamp medical school training to promote this skill. He envisions interns spending 1 month seeing patients without the benefit of reviewing medical histories or chart notes, requiring them to really listen to patients as they talk.

"Another thing about a good doctor is that he shows up," he adds. "My brother-in-law recently had a very serious surgical procedure and after it he developed some complications, including a high fever. His doctor told him to go to the emergency room. He still had problems the next day, but was unable to see his doctor for 4 days."

"Across the street from where I live, a friend of mine was dying in her home. However, no doctor came to visit her. Doctors don't come to visit the dying at home anymore. They call hospice and ambulances. I visited her and spoke with her grandson and her two daughters. They didn't know what to do for her. That is when I wrote an article titled, 'The Doctor Didn't Come.'"

Bob understands the dilemma from the physician's standpoint. "Part of the problem, of course, is economics. There is no compensation for lengthy home visits. It doesn't fit into the present style of medicine for a physician to make a house call and visit for an hour or more. But a good physician should be with the family of a seriously ill or dying patient. He should do this for his own sake as well as the patient's. He needs to go to the river's edge with the patient and not avoid that experience. It has something to do with learning about his mortality as well. No one ever asks a physician about his own sense of mortality and dying. Fortunately, more and more medical schools are beginning to include education about the grief process."

To make his point, Bob shares this story. "I remember the story of a medical student whose father died. She was very attached to her father, went home and stayed with him a month. She was a second or third year student and when she came back to school, she continued giving physicals and taking medical histories in the hospital. A resident who was supervising her reported that she wasn't doing very well. Her memory was lapsing and she seemed to be tired much of the time. The resident supervisor gave her a bad evaluation, forwarding it to a professor. It ended with the resident himself being sent to a class on the nature of mourning. He failed to realize that physicians themselves need to grieve at times. When this oversight occurs, it is a disaster. The doctor who avoids his own emotional situation and does not take care of himself, recognizing his own limits, may end up not being a very good physician."

Bob continues, "Over time I learned to put myself in the patient's shoes and to know whether something was deeply bothering them. This leads me to offering hope, holding hands, and crying at times. I read an article some time ago about the fact that doctors don't cry. I thought to myself, 'Sometimes they do.' I'm not proposing that doctors stand by the bedside and cry every day. But there are times like when a patient is dying or the family is grieving when a few tears from the doctor is not abnormal."

"I have also developed my spiritual self because I know that there is a difference between curing and healing," he says. "I am

so aware and glad that there is a hunger in this area for the majority of my patients. I've taken training in spiritual direction. I hesitate to use the term 'spirituality' because a lot of doctors don't
know what we are speaking about. They think you are some kind
of guru. Spirituality is not in the vocabulary of most physicians.
But ideally what we are attempting to say when using this word
is that we come with love. Each patient is significant. When you
visit with them, it's not just you with your clinical skills. There is
a mystery beyond the clinical arena, the mystery of God. A different kind of power is present. When standing in a hospital room
before a patient, I often feel psychologically naked except for the
fact that I know that God is present. I didn't used to think about
that when I was younger."

*"Invoked or not invoked, God
is present."*

—Carl Jung
Inscription over the entrance
to Jung's home

Expanding on the difference
between curing and healing, Bob
shares his understanding of the power
of healing. "In a recent book written by
the Dalai Lama, he speaks about every
religion focusing attention upon two
basic issues. One is happiness, and the
other is suffering. Ideally, we would
like to have much more happiness than suffering. In the best of all
worlds, there would be no suffering. However, we obviously do
have much suffering and consequently, healing includes the letting
go of the idea of perfectionism. It involves letting go of the idea
that I am immortal and will not suffer. And, certainly in letting go
of one's inflated ego, we let the power of Mystery behind everything in the universe to come forth. Then healing can occur."

"If I am sitting in front of a patient in conversation and if, as a
physician, I can be aware that I too will suffer and am no different
than the patient, then I can be at ease with this suffering patient. I
can let go of the notion that I can cure him or her; I am simply to
be an instrument in the process. As mentioned before, the key is
letting go of perfectionism. The physician must accept his own
imperfect humanity and do the best to control the pain. We have
no control over the outcome in terms of genuine healing; even
death may be a function of healing. It is letting go of the notion
that we must always be doing something, even though all options
have been exhausted. We may be able to cure a particular infection or disease, but we can't cure suffering. When a doctor
embraces this reality, it lifts a great burden from his back and

greatly improves his own well-being. It allows him to listen more intently and show understanding for his or her patients. It is remarkable about how patients react to this. It allows them to accept the fact that they might die, that they have lost their sight, or whatever."

Bob believes that we are currently experiencing a period of transition in medical care. "We are in between the so-called golden age of medicine when physicians monitored themselves and when economics wasn't such a big issue. The physician's role may change. I divide people into two groups, those who 'sit in' and those who 'stick out.' The stick-outs are the creative ones who think up new ways to approach medicine. In this day and age, to be a stick-out is difficult. You are supposed to sort of fit into the system. There have been great philosophers who have said that people who have intuition, passion, and excitement about what they are doing are the ones who get beat down in a system that is closely monitored. For example, there is a list of how you are supposed to treat diabetes and the 'stick-out' has something different in mind. His name will even show up on a computer as a nonconformist, which is too bad because creativity is a major part of medicine."

"However, I think there is a lot of hope that we will transition through this period of physicians being harassed to a time when the ability to speak out and be oneself will be valued. I have hope because in the midst of so many problems in this country, I see an increasing emphasis upon creativity and spirituality. There seems to be a wave of energy emerging, leading us to face the reality that things need to change in society."

"When I visit the University of Washington Medical School and lead a program on care of the dying, I find that the students are wonderful. They seem to be so aware of what's going on and are able to deal with issues in a more comfortable manner than the older doctors. They have so much to offer today in medicine with all of the new advances. Doctors have a tremendous variety of procedures and options. From this standpoint, I think that medicine is going to be different than it has been in the past. There is a whole new approach to treating infections, cancer, diabetes, and so on. For the consumer of medicine, we are going to live longer."

Bob shared a story about John Stanford who, before he died of leukemia, was the beloved superintendent of the Seattle public school system. He was Bob's neighbor, and they were very close friends. In fact, Bob offered a eulogy during his funeral. John was a hero in Seattle and, unfortunately, the hero became ill.

Somewhat sadly, Bob states, "John was a retired military man who engaged in the archetype of the hero. He enjoyed being in charge before and even after stricken with leukemia. The physicians who cared for him treated him as a hero. They even made house calls. Everyone wanted him to live. People described John as a man on a big, white horse with a lance who was going to kill the dragon of cancer. Not only would he conquer the disease, but while in the hospital, he was viewed as someone who could even change the management style of the hospital administrators."

On the other hand, Bob viewed him more as a human being who was quite ill and frightened. John was an Episcopalian, so before entering the hospital, Bob contacted his priest to offer communion. Relatively inactive in terms of his faith, John thought that communion was a last rite rather than the beginning of his healing. "However, the priest and I saw his healing as more of a process of letting go and of knowing that God would take care of him in one way or another."

"As he was dying, for about 3 weeks, John entered a state of semi-unconsciousness, or at least he didn't remember any of the events during that period. Subsequently, when he became more alert, he began to face the reality that his life would not last much longer. He told us that something had changed within him. During this period of semi-unconsciousness, he somehow knew he was no longer in charge and that God was present. Then, before he actually died, he did something quite unusual. He began to write love letters to his wife and his two sons. As an Army officer, he apologized for the many times he was away from the family. The legacy he left to Seattle was to have led and loved the children. However, I told John that he was leaving another legacy, which was that heroes must eventually let go of control and heroism when they die."

Bob shared this story because he believes that healing is not simply curing people of disease. It is rising above death, realizing that there is a greater power, purpose, and mystery involved in the process. We become wiser if we become acquainted with our own humanity and vulnerability. In a way, John Stanford was like St Ignatius who was a military leader before he was wounded and hospitalized. Ignatius' healing journey also caused him to let go of control and embrace his vulnerability, which led to his spiritual transformation.

Bob suggests that such a deep healing process must involve the physician. "Doctors, through Stanford's whole 10-month journey, never let go. John had a 20% chance of surviving to begin with and by the time they got to the second bone marrow transplant, the possibility of recovery dropped to 5%. John experienced deep suffering and went through a great deal of pain attempting to live. Because of his age and the type of leukemia he had, one decision could have been to let him die in a more caring and peaceful manner, or at least in initially engage in a treatment and if that didn't work, to let go of further attempts. Often, the problem with physicians is attempting to maintain life when living is not going to work."

Empathetically, Bob adds, "I'm not being critical of doctors, because I am one and I've done it myself. But you have to ask the question as part of the patient's healing process, just who is healing the doctor? If the doctor is operating as a mere technician and is committed to not letting people die under any circumstances, then what is occurring in that physician's psyche? What are the emotional, social, economic, and spiritual consequences? Everyone suffers along with the patient because no one will let the patient go and say his or her good-byes. People disallow death as part of the healing process."

Bob continues, "Healing is not usually a part of the vocabulary of physicians. As I mentioned earlier, when I was engaged in pastoral care training, the other doctors could not understand what I was doing. And, I felt embarrassed and defensive. Later on, I struggled with these thoughts and feelings, why I was uncomfortable offering only pastoral and not medical care. I was feeling like a powerless fool in a hospital setting where the other doctors knew me. There were some exceptions, when doctors would come to me attempting to understand what I was about, probably because deep within they were uncomfortable with providing only physical care. But this was rare."

"My current thinking is that there are so many blocks to healing. In order to change and to become aware of the greater energies of God in healing, there must be a transformation. People will fight you when you ask them to take their masks off and deal with the nakedness of their humanity and vulnerability. They are deeply afraid of the shadow side of personality. In particular, with the mask of authority of the physician, I believe that power, a sense of immortality, and infallibility are blocks to becoming a doctor of true healing, treating the whole person."

Bob states that he would never speak in these terms to a large body of physicians because most of them would probably either stop listening or simply leave the room. Instead, he would prefer to gather with a few of his physician friends and approach the subject of whole person healing by sharing his personal story. We were delighted to hear these words because it underlines one of the primary reasons why we have written this book. As other physicians seek to take the journey toward transformation, hopefully they will understand that there are companions along the way.

Recovering Workaholic

Jeffrey D. Roth, MD

In writing this book, we attempted to capture something of the heart of each physician's story in its title. We chose "Recovering Workaholic" for Dr Jeffrey Roth partly because the word workaholic probably applies to many physicians. For Jeffrey, other summary descriptors could be "Passionate Engager" or "Slow Grower." When Jim's father was hospitalized this year, about the only time to "catch" (a term used by the nurses) his attending doctor was at 6:30 am or after office hours at 5:30 pm.

We began our interview with Jeffrey, a Chicago-area psychiatrist, by asking him for a few insights into the meaning of "soul." Responding, he talks about soul as some kind of invisible energy connecting us to one another.

"In the past," he confesses, "what has kept me apart from people was the belief that I operated as an individual, alone and self-sufficient. When I give up this idea and accept it as an illusion, I realize how interdependent we are as humans. It is this connection that I identify as soul. Therefore, as a physician, I am most interested in the doctor–patient relationship that is the soul of medicine. As the doctor accepts the responsibility for engaging in the process of caring for another human being, concretely, he or she bonds with soul. I see this as a tangible manifestation of a higher power."

"Thank God I'm not God," he says emphatically. "I believe that by having relationships with people, we create soul and we can do all sorts of things with the soul we create. Some of these things may be useful and some not so helpful. I'm particularly concerned about the fact that sometimes through medical practice we may sell our souls."

The important issue for Jeffrey is to maintain the integrity of relationships with patients, and he is extremely sensitive to anything that intrudes into this affiliation. "This intrusion may be useful or destructive," he explains. "For instance, I maintain a mindfulness about the infringement of insurance companies. When the insurance company enters the picture in one way or another, the doctor–patient relationship as it exists for the purpose of healing may be impaired. This doesn't mean that the insurance company is bad, but it is having an effect. For me, not being able to be honest about this with a patient is unmanageable."

He also believes that anything interfering with the patient–physician relationship impinges upon his passion. For him, passionate energy comes about as a result of connecting intimately with another human being. The bonding creates one of the most intimate relationships existing between people. "Of course, it is not a substitute for personal relationships beyond medicine," he states, "which is one of the traps we physicians can get caught in."

He continues, "One of the damages we have brought upon ourselves with what's called managed care is the idea that there is some virtue in healing people quickly, rather than allowing healing to take place in its own time. Obviously, this is not a very popular idea, especially if it costs more money. I've seen a lot of treatment being done on the premise of saving time; that doesn't particularly work well in terms of the best interests of the patient. Unfortunately, patients are often eager for rapid results as well, because this is the way they have been conditioned by our culture. But," he cautions, "slow growth is good growth."

Reflecting on this statement returns us to Jacob Needleman's insights in his book, *Time and the Soul*. The subtitle of the book is *Where Has All the Meaningful Time Gone . . . and How to Get it Back*.[2] Our obsession with saving time (and money) causes a famine of the soul. If the experience of soul can be linked to connectedness to people (as well as to nature, art, and the like), then we doubt whether it can be rushed. Slow growth is good growth. Slow anything is good for us, whether eating food, walking in the woods, or engaging in sex. Indeed, this may be the underlying message of Thomas Moore as he describes what it means to care for the soul. In his best seller, *The Re-Enchantment of Everyday Life*, Moore writes,

> "Readers of my books have told me over and over: 'I'm too busy to care for my soul.' If we are indeed too busy, then it's obvious that we need to relax, to learn how to do less and behold more, to become lazy in the soul instead of hyperactive in the spirit." [3]

With all of its efficiency standards, this could be the essential problem of managed care; it prematurely forces us to reengage in

---

[2] Needleman J. *Time and the Soul: Where Has All the Meaningful Time Gone?…and How to Get It Back*. New York, NY: Currency/Doubleday; 1998.
[3] Moore T. *The Re-Enchantment of Everyday Life*. New York, NY: HarperCollins; 1996: 357.

a busy life and contributes to famine of the soul. *Slow healing is soul healing!*

In the midst of health care's accelerating change and its ensu-ing stress, the importance of caring for oneself emotionally and spiritually has been underlined by a number of physicians. Concurring, Jeffrey says, "The first thing I had to learn is that I can't take care of myself in isolation. In this respect, I am grateful that there is actually a model for psychiatrists to take care of themselves. For psychiatrists to seek their own care is at least somewhat acceptable today as a professional norm. When I became interested in addiction treatment, I began working with a number of others who, in the process of their personal recovery, recognized that they needed a support group. When I saw what they did, I decided to join Al-Anon, which is a support group for the family and friends of alcoholics. It was the first experience I had of really letting go of compulsively held individual identity and of workaholism. With physicians, I've heard it called the 'M.Diety syndrome.' Often, one of the problems of the family and friends of alcoholics is that they want to assume responsibility for and control someone else's drinking. It was very helpful for me to hear this and to recognize that this is something I am also capable of doing. However, that would rob me of participation in a rela-tionship with a patient."

"I learned that it is not my job to fix the problem, a critically important realization. I had heard this intellectually in medical school, but had not integrated it emotionally. Ambroise Paré, the French surgeon, said 'I dressed him; and God healed him.' In other words, I may say something to a patient, but whether it is received or has an impact upon him or her is not up to me. Of course, a lot depends upon how we have built a relationship with one another."

Ambroise Paré was a sixteenth century military surgeon. At that time, gunshot wounds were classified as contused, burned, and poisoned. They were cauterized with a red-hot iron or hot oil, leading to enormous pain. On one occasion, not having sufficient oil, Paré applied ointment and bandaged the wounds, greatly improving the treatment.

Paré often is described as a gentle doctor with a deep belief that human lives are worth saving. This attitude probably emerged from his devout faith. Expanding upon Paré's perceptive statement "I dressed him, and God healed him," Sherwin Nuland, MD, writes, "Things are no different today. Whether determined by God or nature, there is a point in the process of healing past which no physician can take a patient." [4]

Jeffrey began his journey in medicine with an eye toward winning a Nobel Prize for the cure of cancer. Laughing at himself when he recalls the goal, he becomes serious as he explains why he selected medicine and in particular psychiatry.

"I was going to be an oncologist performing some clinical work but mostly performing outstanding research. Back in high school, I worked with an oncologist. During summer vacations from Yale, I worked in this field at the University of Rochester. Becoming a physician was supposed to be a stepping stone to the research."

"However, an essential turning point in my career came during a clerkship in internal medicine. One Monday morning, I was making rounds with a female intern who had been trained at Mt. Sinai. She was presenting a patient whom she had admitted the evening before, a young, black male who was a heroin addict and who had medical complications. Tired and obviously upset, she introduced the patient to us and to the resident doctor she was working with as 'this 24-year-old black piece of shit.' This experience colored the entire next 6 weeks of my clerkship."

It is obvious that these deeply disturbing experiences still rankle him, and he continues. "There were also a number of patients called 'GOMERS,' which I learned was an acronym for 'get them out of my emergency room.' *(Note: We are told that other acronyms include GORK [patients with serious neurological damage] and SHPOS [for subhuman piece of shit]).* Many of these people were old and poor, with a limited ability to communicate or express feelings. And, at that time, my job as a medical student was to learn how to perform invasive procedures on people who had very limited ability to communicate; it was assumed they would die."

"I was confronted with what today I can view as the nightmare of medicine," he states matter-of-factly. "Up until that time, I was in total denial that it existed. Medical education was almost a 100% technological experience, very alienating at a time when I was very lonely to begin with. It devastated me. I did have a few patients whom I was able to connect with, and I was grateful for that, but it didn't seem to have anything to do with the practice of medicine. I treated them for various medical problems, but I was most inter-

---

[4] Nuland S. *Doctors, The Biography of Medicine.* New York, NY: Alfred A. Knopf; 1988: 107.

ested in speaking with them and finding out about their lives. Until then, I didn't realize that this was such a great interest."

Jeffrey's very next rotation was in psychiatry. During it, he witnessed physicians who were talking to patients and who were willing to engage with them. So, during the course of the year, he shifted his interests in that direction, eventually doing his residency in this specialty. His interest in research receded, helped along by the fact that there was little psychiatric research money available in the 1980s. So, he entered private practice.

Jeffrey especially emphasizes his interest in working with groups of people. "By working with groups, my early insights that we are really not insolated individuals emerged. We can learn in groups how people connect with one another in ways that sometimes are explicit and sometimes not."

His path ultimately led to an interest in treating addictions. As he recalls, "I was involved in some consulting at a community hospital and subsequently was invited to be the medical director in the alcohol abuse unit. I told them I was interested if I could meet with the patients in groups. They looked at me as though I had come from Mars. Why would a psychiatrist want to spend more than just a few minutes with any patient? The previous doctor would simply visit with someone for a minute or so, write a note, and collect his per diem for the visit. But I wasn't interested in that kind of medicine. I wanted to learn something about people's experiences and the best way to gain this insight was to work with groups. For a psychiatrist, this was an unheard of concept. But I did this for a year and this is where I learned about the notion of powerlessness and the process of recovery. This is what led me to an interest in treating addictions."

Jeffrey believes that healing involves the process of engaging in a relationship and it takes place through the recovery of one's soul. It is the process of connection that heals. When we let go of what we have been doing that is killing us and attach to something that is constructive, healing happens. Believing that spirituality is a part of the process, he describes spirituality as a belief in the existence of a power greater than oneself. It could also be described as the route toward finding meaning in one's life. We cannot find any meaning for ourselves without some kind of connection beyond ourselves. In addition, he affirms, "With respect to our relationship with other people, we likely cannot see things about ourselves that others can see."

Among the lessons Jeffrey learned from the 12-step program is a very simple understanding of prayer and meditation. Amplifying on this belief he states, "Prayer is the process of talking to God and meditation is our way of listening to God. For me, God is not an abstract concept. God exists in the relationship. So, when I am telling my story it is a form of prayer and when I am learning something from other people I experience it as a meditative event."

"God is a not a place – but a moment. When two people act in a truly human fashion, God fills the space between them . . . "

—Martin Buber

Jeffrey does not routinely discuss such thoughts with his colleagues. He says, "I share what I experience when it is asked of me. Give me a platform and I'll talk! However, I am mindful of the possibility of promoting rather than attracting. I don't wish to promote in the sense of adopting a proselytizing mode, because it would be harmful to me. Some of my colleagues seem very open to discussing spirituality, while others would not be interested. If a physician shares a particular problem with me, I like to be able to identify with that person and share my own experience. During that dialogue, I will live my orientation and not preach it. In any engagement, remaining focused upon the present moment is very important to me. Some people actively guard against discussions having a spiritual overtone and it is not my wish to press the issue."

"He who teaches a child is as if he created it."

—The Talmud

In Jeffrey's opinion, physicians who seem to be connected to soul exhibit several specific characteristics. The first is *curiosity* and, surprisingly, along with that is the notion of *playfulness*. He explains, "I experience soul coming from our connection to the little kid inside of us. One of the challenges for me is to be a professional physician and to be a little kid at the same time. It involves the ability to identify compassionately with the people I am treating and recognizing that we all have a childlike heritage. Being curious for me includes the notion that children possess a natural, unfettered, inquisitive bent. They often pursue their interests in what might seem a relentless fashion to adults. They are not necessarily being compulsive, but do it in the service of being engrossed. They wish to understand and to feel, to hold and be held."

Jeffrey continues, "Therefore, as a physician, it means psychologically, emotionally, spiritually, and sometimes physically, holding another person. We can hold a hand and we can hold a particular feeling. So we say, 'Yes, I hear you feeling sad.' It's not a computer-generated feeling because I may have had the same experience myself at times. We can laugh, cry, and be angry together. For me, this is what it means to be connected to soul and having a healing relationship with another person."

Both inside as well as outside of the practice of medicine, Jeffrey enhances his life and sense of well-being by letting go of the disease of workaholism. He maintains, "It is every bit as deadly as alcohol would be to an alcoholic. It involves not abstaining from work, but finding a way to not work compulsively."

He declares, "For me, having boundaries around my work is very important. I have many activities in my life that are not work. Of course, being in intimate personal relationships is very important. I also have hobbies and interests vital to experiencing aliveness. For example, I like to roller blade," he confesses grinning. "It brings out my little kid. I can roller blade in a way that becomes joyful play or that results in compulsive work, and I don't always know the difference."

Being a workaholic is one of the most important lessons learned throughout his life. He says emphatically, "I'm a workaholic. If I forget it, I'm going to begin working compulsively again. If I remember it, I'll have lots of time and energy in my life to do other things. I don't ever expect *not* to be a recovering workaholic. If I start working compulsively again, I will be a workaholic in denial."

"My sponsor in Al-Anon, who helps with my recovery program from workaholism, taught me how to play golf. I had to commit to not keeping score in order to enjoy the game. I also had to let go of the notion that I had to take lessons. People were telling me that, in order to play the game, you had to take instruction. But I knew that if I began taking lessons, I would become obsessed with my golf score. I wanted to enjoy the game and not try to be another Tiger Woods."

As mentioned before, Jeffrey joined Al-Anon initially because he wanted to learn from the experience. Today, he claims to have gone full circle and readily admits that, like most if not all of us, he has had, and probably will continue to have, setbacks both in his personal life and in his career.

Sadly he shares, "A major storm came when our first child was diagnosed as being autistic. Living with someone who has a serious disease has been my most significant challenge. It is a matter of realizing that there is nothing I can do about it. He became more and more disruptive in our household, to the point where we found a residential facility for him when he was 12. That left a tremendous hole in our home."

"That was in 1996 and about a year later I faced a second major setback. My wife told me that she didn't love me anymore. Through 20/20 hindsight, I realized that it had been coming for a long period of time. When we were married, we bought into the assumption that we would remain the same persons throughout our lives. However, through my work, my recovery from workaholism, and my personal growth, I betrayed that assumption by changing my behavior, resulting in a changed relationship."

In his book, *Synchronicity*,[5] Joseph Jaworski reports about returning home one evening only to be confronted with those same words, "I don't love you any more," and the fact that his wife had found another man. We wonder how often these words really express the truth about a situation. Perhaps more appropriately and truthfully would be to say, "I don't want you as my father (mother, provider, caretaker, etc) anymore because I have found (or need to find) another father (mother, provider, caretaker)." A shift in one person's behavior may cause a crisis for another person.

Continuing, Jeffrey says, "The slowness of the divorce process has actually helped me to grieve and to appreciate how important grieving is as a spiritual process. You have to feel the sadness, anger, and hurt that not only came about because of the divorce, but also because of the loss of my son as a more ordinary adolescent."

Jeffrey acknowledges obvious disruptions in his practice resulting from the divorce. His patients eventually sensed his sadness and loneliness and, in dutiful fashion, tried to fix him, typical behavior for "good" addicts. He says, "As part of my practice, I work with a number of impaired physicians. I see how a physician's impairment can hold him or her away from practicing in the full interest of a patient. They tend to become rigid and keep a distance from others, but mostly they are destructive to themselves. Because I have seen this behavior in others, it became very important for me not to react to my loneliness by keeping such a distance or by using my patients as a substitute for what I was losing."

---

[5] Jaworski J. *Synchronicity: The Inner Path of Leadership*. San Francisco, CA: Berrett-Koehler; 1996.

It was also during this period in his life when he experienced two disheartening and wounding occurrences. Acknowledging the pain of that time, he explains. "Previously, I never had any complaints about me professionally, but during the course of a year there were two of them. It was difficult, and there were times when I contemplated what I would call professional suicide. In distress, I began listening to the 2 voices of patients that were critical of me instead of the 60 voices of patients and friends who served as my cheerleaders. Listening to the critical inner voice, I thought to myself that perhaps I should simply close up the shop. I call that professional suicide. Why would I want to give up this incredibly joyful environment? Fortunately, I had been trained in my personal recovery process well enough to get a lot of help from other friends and professionals. That is what got me through the ordeal."

Jeffrey's passion for medicine becomes abundantly clear when listening to him. He is also optimistic about the medical profession, stating, "My vision is that medicine has been going through its own addiction. There was a point in the past, probably in the early 1900s, where the doctor–patient relationship was sacred. Also, some really great things were happening in terms of technology. But with the growth of technology, a number of obstacles developed that tended to undermine the doctor–patient relationship. Technology and economics together began to eat away at soulful medicine. To the extent that we physicians have become preoccupied with these things more than the practice of patient care, we become diseased in the basic meaning of the term. It's not a terminal illness, but something we can recover from."

"Managed care is to medicine as Antabuse is to alcoholism. Antabuse causes the alcoholic to vomit when drinking, and I suspect that many doctors view managed care in this way. But, I believe we are moving in a positive direction; if we are able to recover together and get back in touch with the soul of medicine, then technology and money and managed care will no longer be such a drain of energy. We must give technology a place second to humanity. The same is true about the need for money. It is important, but only in a subordinate role."

After the interview, we reflected on the difference between calling and compulsion. Perhaps, as James Hillman maintains, calling springs from an inborn pattern of interests and skills, the soul's code (as discussed in the Introduction to this book). More than anything else, it leads us to the joy of play. Compulsion erupts from a more extrinsic desire to be needed, admired, respected, or controlling, often leading to frustration and failure. For many of us, the courage is to take the road less traveled to our true passion.

Light From an Angel

Nancy Huet Neubauer, MD

Six months before our interview, Dr Nancy Neubauer and her family moved from Portland, Oregon, to Whidbey Island, Washington. She and her husband, Larry, reached this point in their lives because of a trauma and, as we shall find, the light from an angel.

Nancy and her husband Larry were living the so-called good life. The parents of two children, they had a full-time nanny, many friends, and a busy schedule. She was entrenched in a successful career as a radiologist in an academic center. He also was enjoying a successful career in medical physics, involving significant travel. For both of them, success was defined by being in demand, enjoying their children, and by engaging in all of the trappings of their active life. Their only big question was, "Have we arrived?"

"Our busy lifestyle provided us with value and importance," Nancy recalls, "yet we were consciously aware of depths not reached. It came to light when our 2-year-old daughter, Audrey, was diagnosed as having kidney cancer. On Thanksgiving evening in 1999, I felt a mass in her abdomen, and being a radiologist, I took her to the hospital to do an ultrasound. This escalated into a formal diagnosis of a fairly advanced cancer (Wilms' tumor). Her right kidney and several lymph nodes had to be removed. On her third birthday, she received her first chemotherapy treatment."

"As you can imagine," she continues, "this changed us forever. Although the experience has been overwhelming, it brings us many gifts. It forced us out of the box of our daily routine. This crisis shifted everything for us. We developed so much more clarity about what choices are important in life. I took several months off from work, and then my husband quit his job."

"As serendipity would have it, at the beginning of the crisis, I received a phone call from the Radia Imaging Group, informing me of an available job on Whidbey island directing a radiology program. I knew from a friend that the island was a pastoral setting with much to offer. The call came when I was in intensive care with my daughter and I disregarded it. Then, about 6 weeks later, I heard again from Radia and was ready to listen."

When Nancy and her husband visited the island, they again experienced a feeling of synchronicity, feeling a tug pulling them in this direction. For many years, they had talked about living in a more rural environment, living a simpler life with less complicated choices. After conducting research on the area, they ultimately made the decision to relocate.

"We love it here," Nancy says enthusiastically, her eyes sparkling. She describes the island as a nurturing place and the community as being open and welcoming. Living on a 5-acre farm offers an opportunity to have animals. Today, they board one horse and lease another and plan to expand that number. After our interview, Nancy will take a horseback-riding lesson. And, next spring, they will put in a garden and raise chickens.

Today, the intention is for both of them to work part time, Nancy as a radiologist and her husband as a medical physics consultant. Their goal is to stay directed and balanced, not letting work carry them away from life.

"My daughter is one of my heroes," Nancy states softly. "She possesses an incredible spirit and remains so in love with life. She glows, even throughout chemotherapy as all of her hair fell out. She draws our attention to what we value most in our lives."

"She went through treatment as well as could be expected. If you are going to grow a solid organ tumor as a pediatric patient, this one is a good one to grow. While her disease was advanced and the rate of reoccurrence is high, her ultimate prognosis remains favorable. Either way, we will face the situation with courage in our hearts."

As Audrey went through her chemotherapy treatment, the family developed an agenda to care for her, making sure she kept her strength up and taking her to the hospital every Friday, or anytime she had a fever. "When the treatment came to an end and they removed the catheter, we went home that night feeling really weird," Nancy remembers. "We felt out of control, but then it made us aware that while having an agenda and a focus, nonetheless, we never were in charge of the situation.

Ultimately," she believes, "control is an illusion. Mortality and death teach us to live in the moment and to love openly. So, in a really good way, the experience impacted us profoundly."

Nancy states that, before this experience, she held an underlying fear and anxiety of such a diagnosis. Because she worked in pediatric radiology at the academic center in Portland, she was around children with devastating diagnoses. "I often wondered how families could muster courage," she exclaimed. "I used to think about it quite often. I found a lot of amazement and wonder in how people gained the strength to deal with these problems. What would I do if it had been my child? When it did happen to us, I was grateful for my medical knowledge, but soon learned not to be a doctor to my child. I knew I was out of control and I let that happen. I didn't have competing agendas. My role became to support my daughter and the rest of my family."

Nancy's son, Grant, is a sensitive, mature 9 year old. He has spent a lot of time around adults and even participated in some of Nancy's residency activities. When Audrey was diagnosed, Grant required more information. He knew of "cancer" and needed to understand it within the context of his own family.

"We were very honest about the situation, never attempting to protect him from the trauma," she asserts. "We rocked his boat with all of the changes. We continue to spend a lot of time talking to both of our children about the values and challenges in our daily life."

We asked Nancy how the events of the past year impacted her practice as a radiologist. "My training taught me to be scientific and objective. The message is that I am the physician with the knowledge and you are the patient with a diagnosis. Although I would be compassionate with patients, I sometimes felt distanced. However, during this recent role reversal with Audrey, I really came to understand there is so much less of a separation between a physician and a patient. The only division between us is this little bit of knowledge I have. Ultimately we still need to be very connected, much in the same way that I am linked to my family and friends. Today, even if it is a brief moment, I feel more engaged."

"Mutuality in all things,
isolation in none,
That is the natural law."

—O.S. Fowler
Creative and Sexual Science
(1870)

Nancy comments that the other thing she has learned to do is relinquish her ego as she nears the age of 40. "People in medicine tend to be type 'A' perfectionists," she claims. "Today, I see myself as a recovering perfectionist. When consulting with patients and with other doctors, I no longer portray myself as someone with all of the answers. I like to think I have more humility."

We see a relationship between humility and spirituality, and asked Nancy about the latter. She replies, "Spirituality is very personal. I feel very vulnerable when I engage in discussions about it.

I was raised in a fairly nonreligious family. I saw my father as a very spiritual person, but we didn't attend church. During my high school years, I somehow felt I was cheated in this respect. I felt that I lacked a formal grounding in spirituality so I attended a Catholic college in search of this structure."

Smiling, she continues, "Today, I'm probably also a recovering Catholic, but see myself as more of a spiritual person than ever before. I certainly try to be less judgmental, accepting my own journey and that of others, learning as I go."

Nancy acknowledges praying for her patients. Understandably, she connects prayer to the grieving process. "We are trained in medicine to be scientifically objective. We take in information, make a diagnosis, and come up with a treatment plan. Emotion can be viewed as a weakness. However, it is unreal to be objective all of the time. I can privately express grief and anguish through prayer. Prayer is a powerful tool, allowing me to remain connected to the humanity of difficult situations with patients. Obviously, such expressions must be offered only when appropriate, but if grief isn't expressed in some manner, it's not going to go away."

"In this respect, as a doctor, allowing oneself to stay connected on a human level while still providing quality medical care is a crucial combination. Our formal medical training provides us with a scientific structure. We cultivate compassion through our own experience. Most patients desire this compassionate, holistic approach to medicine. It makes the relationship between doctor and patient more believable and realistic."

When asked about what experiences led her into medicine, Nancy talked about the older, childless German couple—both physicians—who lived next to her home as she was growing up. Starting at about the age of 8, Dr Jonnen Kalb would grab her hand, kiss her, and say, "Nancy, you are so smart; someday you will be a doctor." It must have influenced her.

In college, she liked science and took a course in chemistry (her father was a chemist). She declares, "I fell in love with the professors in this department, convincing myself that I would be a PhD biochemist. It became my college major and was followed by additional studies at the University of Chicago. Working in the laboratory was not fulfilling, so I ended my studies. I followed the advice of my physician neighbors and applied to medical school."

Medicine engages Nancy's passion in the sense of being able to connect with people. She declares, "There are parts of medicine that I love and parts that I hate. I love understanding physiology and anatomy, learning new ways to make diagnoses. However, I struggle with the ethical conflicts. We are always gaining new knowledge and making technical progress, but I question the bigger picture as a society. Are we always attempting to postpone or escape death? We expand choices just to escape the final outcome of life."

"During the past few years, my husband and I have been participating in a medical mission project in Honduras. Specifically, we have been establishing a diagnostic imaging center, with an emphasis upon breast examinations and treatments. We set up the facility, provide equipment and sustainable education for doctors and technologists. I feel very fortunate to provide this assistance. Honduras is a very poor and devastated country. I take away more than I give to these people. They exude such an appreciation for life because they are not afraid of death, not the way we are in North America. Our society pathologically views life as linear, forgetting the entire life cycle. Those people face death on almost a daily basis, empowering them to live more fully and appreciate life. They end up being so grateful for the little, simpler things in life and are probably richer because of it."

_____

"The call to simplicity and freedom is a reminder that our worth comes not from the amount of our involvements, achievements, or possessions, but from the depth and care which we bring to each moment, place, and person in our lives."

— Richard A. Bower
Living Simply (1981)

Earlier in our interview, Nancy called medical training a very disruptive process. We asked her to expand upon that statement. "Speaking only from my own experience," she answers, "you enter medical school with such high ideals, but the process becomes a knowledge exchange for your soul. I know there is a desire to make it more compassionate, but there is so much information and technical data you need to take into a practice. You become so exhausted. You may even become physically and financially distraught. In addition, the emotional impact is often tremendous because of suffering, loss, and mistakes. In general, most people neither have the time nor tools to process their experiences. I've seen a lot of people enter medical school idealistic and emerge cynical, angry, and judgmental. We ultimately find ourselves expected to be nurturing, yet medical school is not a nurturing place. But, I don't have an answer for it," she says shaking her head.

For Nancy, the word *soul* signifies compassion for self and others. It involves uncovering the truth inside of us. She finds soul being challenged by our insecurities, expectations, and judgments. "However," she reports, "if we can free ourselves from these elements, we can become so much more alive and compassionate. Soul includes being aware of the connectedness of all of life."

Along these lines, Nancy hopes that, throughout her life, people will view her as someone who approached them with an open heart. "My personal goal," she informs us, "is to always live with compassion for everyone, including myself. Self-compassion frees us to be present with the needs of others."

Concluding the interview, Nancy declares, "When I saw your questions, I thought it was a great opportunity to stop and really think about my choice of medicine as a career and to assess my life in general. One of the questions you asked involved having a favorite poem or quotation. I often find quotes which resonate inside. I recently read a quote that Dan Millman used in his book, *Living on Purpose*: 'We are each angels with only one wing. We fly only by embracing one another.'" (By Luciano de Crescenzo).

Then, Nancy told this story about one such angel. "Three days after Audrey was diagnosed with the kidney tumor, she underwent surgery to remove the tumor and place an indwelling central venous catheter. She was monitored for 2 days in the intensive care unit prior to being transferred to the oncology ward to initiate radiation therapy and chemotherapy. My husband and I felt both terrified and overwhelmed. We were sitting at Audrey's bedside when we saw the first bright light. Open popped the door and in walked a gregarious 9-year-old girl, bald from chemotherapy with a big scar across the top of her head. She wore blue, oversized glasses; floppy slippers; and an enormous smile. She said, 'Hi!' Then she walked straight over to Audrey, asking her name and quizzing us about her problem. We explained that Audrey had just had a kidney removed, to which the little girl responded, 'Well, I had a brain tumor. I had my operation back in August.'"

"The girl informed us that she lived in Bend, Oregon, returning to the hospital on a monthly basis for 5 days of treatment. The first thing she would routinely do after checking in was to make rounds on all of the children on the oncology ward. So she visited with us and we were captivated. For the first time we let go of our own preoccupations. 'I had surgery 8 months ago, started chemotherapy, and lost all of my hair. But that's okay, because it will grow back and be long and curly again.'"

"She began to describe the 3-hour trip from her home to the hospital, saying, 'The drive is so beautiful. The sun reflected off the mountains. My dad and I played music and talked and laughed together. I love to come here because my dad and I talk to each other the whole way. And aren't the nurses here just great?'"

"She was so animated. Her eyes danced. My husband and I were mesmerized to the point of being unable to speak. A light emanated from her whole being as she told all the stories. I know from her diagnosis that, today, her chance for survival is low."

"As she walked out the door, suddenly for both of us, all of the lights went on. This is what living is all about. It is why we live, not so we can reach 80 years old when we die, but so we can be present and live each day fully. After this experience, our perspective shifted. The joy and animation that we witnessed in our young visitor modeled the courage and grace we would need to face the unknown. She must be an angel."

Medicine Man

Gary Olbrich, MD

His work funded in part by the Tennessee Medical Foundation, Gary Olbrich, MD, serves as medical director of the Physicians Health Program (PHP) for that state. He explains that the purpose of the PHP is "to protect patients from identifiably impaired physicians and to afford impaired physicians every opportunity to be rehabilitated to productive medical practice." In addition to chemical dependence, and mental or emotional illness, the program has been expanded in the 1990s to assist physicians and their families with a wider range of problems, which include dealing with rage, getting along in cooperative fashion with other group practice members, and focusing other psychosocial issues that inhibit a physician's ability to practice the healing arts.

Gary's office is located in the rear of his home in southern Nashville. The drive through this historic Forest Hill section appeals to the senses. Named after Southern heroes like Robert E. Lee and Oliver Cromwell, the streets coil their way through wooded hills, along stone fences, and past large, colonial-style church buildings.

Providing physician assistance care for some 10 years is Gary's second career. Previously he practiced internal medicine in small communities, working virtually 24 hours a day, 7 days a week. A motorcycle accident that should have taken his life contributed to a later dependency on alcohol.

The burnout Gary experienced fairly early in his career added to his addictive problems, until he finally entered a number of treatment programs. Gary attributes the 12-step program associated with Alcoholics Anonymous as what finally carried him through the process of healing. "The real key to it was spirituality," he believes. "The 12-step program evokes a spiritual journey."

Gary is part Cherokee Indian. His father's work in the oil fields of Oklahoma required the family to move around every few years. As a child, Gary had serious trauma in his life (he suspects this is true of many physicians). He found establishing friendships only to leave them every few years to be emotionally devastating. But, there was little or nothing he could do about it, so he sublimated the pain and then began developing his role of a caretaker of others. More importantly, he confesses that he wanted power and control over his life. "I wanted to live the way I wanted to live and to move only if I wanted to move. I figured I could best achieve such independence by becoming a doctor. I also wanted the prestige of being respected as a physician in the community."

Gary believes that if he had it to do over again, he would still become a physician, but not in any sense of fitting into a traditional model. "Actually, what I am doing now is the most soul-satisfying thing I have ever done. This is my passion; today I am much more of a teacher."

Gary finds the world of medicine today a different reality contributing to the angst that some physicians are feeling. "More and more doctors are seeking our services because they are angry and frustrated. They can't change the system that works against their practices, so they must resort to changing themselves. And, these are not simply isolated individuals. I am currently working with two physician groups and an entire medical department of a medical school. With this latter group, people simply cannot communicate and are at each other's throats."

He continues, "Doctors feel trapped and live with the perception that they cannot do anything else vocationally. They are highly trained in their professions, and it doesn't really prepare them for anything else." However, working for many years as a career development specialist with highly trained professionals in a number of disciplines, Jim believes this is more of an assumption than a reality. Multigifted physicians are intelligent, reliable, adaptable, and maintain high levels of energy. Their skills may include leadership, problem-solving/creativity, teamwork, manual dexterity, caring and instructing, public contact, and physical stamina. Physicians are able to learn, work hard for long periods of time, and make decisions under stress.

According to Suzanne Fraker, Director, Product Line Development, AMA Press,

"There is more opportunity . . . away from the bedside than ever before. Physicians are among the most capable individuals in the workforce, and their particular training in the biomedical and clinical sciences makes them a valuable asset to law firms, businesses, consulting firms, and other corporations."

Health care is a very diverse field; most physicians might not realize how many opportunities are available and how they are expanding in the general health care arena.

Sometimes vocational passion emerges from tragic life experiences, which certainly holds true for Gary Olbrich. "My vocational passion is trying to prevent some of the tragedies that occurred in my life from happening to other physicians," he states. "When I started on my journey to get well in 1982, there weren't programs available like the PHP. There especially were no structured programs for doctors who desired to reenter their practices and survive."

The 2000 AMA International Conference titled, "Recapturing the Soul of Medicine, " reinforced his passion of helping physicians in reclaiming the soul of medicine. He believes this reclamation means identifying and pursuing meaning in life and vocation. As he says, "I personally got so caught up in the technical part of critical care medicine that I lost touch with the human contact. I lost sight of why I went into medicine in the first place."

In 2000, Gary began conducting a series of seminars in an effort to encourage physicians to develop a sense of recapturing soul and to learn how to care for each other. Unfortunately, few physicians have moved past what one physician calls the "John Wayne syndrome," the belief that it is a sign of weakness to admit such a need. Gary is convinced that, "If there is any hope for physicians, it must come from the inside." He frequently refers to a book written in 1904 by Sir William Osler, MD, titled *Aequanimitas*. [6] In addition to being a pioneer in medical education, Osler was a real humanist and spent a large part of his later life adapting humanism to medicine. He spoke of the united, worldwide profession of doctoring as having done more in the nineteenth century for mankind than any other group of people. "United is the key word," says Gary. "Unless physicians can find a common purpose and become collegial again, I don't see any light at the end of the tunnel. They will not be able to recapture the nobility and soul of the profession."

He tells us that, unfortunately, very few opportunities exist for building community among physicians. It is a major problem. In Tennessee, the PHP organized a number of groups across the state called Caduceus Groups. Originally established for physicians only, any health care professional can participate. These groups meet weekly and are self-led. In addition to providing a safe place for sharing and support, they are designed to help the participants

---

[6] Osler W. *Aequanimitas*. Philadelphia, PA: The Blakiston Company; 1932.

move from impairment (of any kind) to becoming more completely whole, human, and healed. Gary notes that, "Because of all the moaning about medicine these days, doctors tend not to go to lunch with their peers or even to society meetings. In addition, because of the 'big brother' reporting mechanism and the concerns over medical errors, there is hardly any place to let your hair down. Because they have learned to take care of everyone else and have not developed many self-help skills, they have become terribly isolated."

Gary suggests that the most difficult issue in working with impaired physicians is that they hardly have any idea of who they are apart from being a practitioner. He says that chemically dependent physicians are almost fortunate that they are afflicted with the disease because they are sometimes sent away for 3 or 4 months. This is an intense program of study. It is almost like getting a PhD in "Who am I?" Many of them have no clue as to how other people perceive them and how they impact other persons. "So many doctors are human doers rather than human beings."

Gary believes that another critical element in reclaiming the soul of medicine revolves around the way it is being taught in many schools. "Unfortunately, the shaming, demeaning, and desocializing approach to education is still in place a lot more than we care to admit. The general attitude of some professors is that 'if it was good enough for me, it is good enough for today's students.'" Regrettably, physicians come out of this environment being emotionally numb and cynical.

"Darth Vadar (in Star Wars) has not developed his own humanity. He's a robot. He's a bureaucrat, living not in terms of himself but in terms of an imposed system. This is the threat to our lives that we all face today. Is the system going to flatten you out and deny your humanity?"

—Joseph Campbell
The Power of Myth (1988)

Gary contends that, however it is described, we are all born with a soul and that it is not something we need to create. "Soul is the life force making us human. It serves as the bridge between intellectual intelligence and emotional intelligence." As such, he believes that healing comes from within. As most physicians know as a result of the placebo effect, one's mental perception and sense of purpose have an enormous impact on health. During his recovery process from alcohol impairment, Gary, who, as mentioned, is part Cherokee Indian, reclaimed part of the power of having purpose through a return to his Native American heritage. "I didn't realize it at the time, but when I was a boy playing cowboys and Indians, I always wanted to be an Indian," he remembers. Especially during recovery, he gravitated toward expressions and experiences of soul within his personal heritage and studied such Native American symbolism as the medicine wheel.

The Native Americans viewed the medicine wheel as a magic, quadrated circle symbolizing the entire world. They saw life as a circle, from birth to death to rebirth, representing totality or wholeness. It is quadrated because the number 4 is seen as being numerically complete as in the four corners of the earth or the four seasons in nature. Gary's study of the medicine wheel undoubtedly was and is part of his journey to recapture the original purpose of medical practice and to center him in its comprehensive energy.

Gary concluded our visit by sharing a phenomenal experience that happened to him when he was a senior medical student at Stanford. "I had been fascinated by many of the chronically ill patients, some of whom would say to me, 'I'm going to die.' There were days when I knew what the patient was speaking about and could predict the outcome. He or she would, in fact, pass away. This ability to intuit an event really scared me and I have not shared these experiences with people until recently. It scared me so much that I stopped making such predictions."

Gary suggests that some people have *the will to live*, which Arnold Hutschnecker speaks about in his book by the same title. [7] Other people decide to die and are at peace with this decision. When a physician is sometimes able to intuit such a will, we suspect they may be connected to the force of the second serpent in the caduceus, which again as Jacob Needleman suggests, is moving back toward union with the Source.

---

[7] Hutschnecker A. *The Will to Live*. New York, NY: Cornerstone Library; 1978.

Physician's Helper

Lynn Hankes, MD

Dr Lynn Hankes serves as the director of the Washington Physicians Health Program as well as current president of the Federation of State Physician Health Programs. The dual roles are close to his heart. He began our conversation by discussing the programs before talking personally.

"Physician Health Programs (PHPs) used to be confined primarily to dealing with chemical dependency," he explains. "Over the years, they began to incorporate pure mental illness, mostly helping physicians with affective disorders of one kind or another. They began to flourish as medical boards and the medical community at large saw some merit in a more proactive approach, allowing programs to conduct their work under the umbrella of confidentiality. There were exponential increases in the number of doctors whom we could help. As a subpopulation of people with the disease of alcoholism, physicians have the best successful outcomes, in excess of 85%. Some PHPs began to provide services for compulsive gambling, psychosexual disorders, stress, and the difficult/disruptive doctor."

We were curious about Lynn's background, how he became interested in medicine and ultimately what led to his current passion. "My only exposure to the medical profession as a child," he recalls, "was in my father's drugstore. My father enjoyed business development. A high school buddy of his went to pharmacy school, and in the mid-forties, my Dad financed his opening of a drug store in Aurora, Illinois. I was 10 years old and putting prescription bottles in racks and stocking shelves. Doctors visited the store from time to time and that was my first exposure to medicine. Dad's grand plan for me was to attend the University of Notre Dame, major in economics, then gain an MBA degree and some experience in a large organization. I would eventually join him in running his empire of five businesses. At the time, I wanted to major in philosophy, but that didn't compute for him."

"Then a strange thing happened to me which I believe in retrospect was not a coincidence. In the summer between my junior and senior years of college, my father was out of town and I received an urgent phone call from my mother. My brother's playmate injured his hand while at our house and was taken to the emergency room, bleeding like a stuffed pig. As the family hero, I went to the emergency room to check on the boy. The physician involved was Dr Eugene Balthazar, a classic, old-time general practitioner who also performed many surgeries. He asked if I would like to observe him sewing up the boy's hand. Being curious, I said I would. I got through the first part okay when he injected a local anesthetic. Blood dripped all over the place and the kid was screaming. When the anesthetic took hold, all of a sudden things got calm. About midway through the procedure, I began to feel queasy and excused myself, went out into the alley and vomited. Attempting to maintain a façade of 'Mr. Cool,' I returned to watch the end of the procedure. I was fascinated with the whole thing."

"Then, the doctor asked whether I would like to witness a real operation. I said, 'Oh, wow!' He invited me to come to the hospital to see a cesarean section. The next morning I'm standing off to the side watching this miraculous event occurring. I was not only fascinated, but also perceived it as a meaningful and purposeful event. Dr Balthazar soon became my hero. I followed him around all summer, watching him deliver babies and perform other procedures. Observing medical procedures was not a problem back in the 1950s," he quickly points out. "I came to find out later that I was not his only protégé. He was, in fact, always recruiting for the medical profession."

"The life of every man [and woman] is a diary in which he means to write one story and writes another."

—J.M. Barrier

Recalling his reluctance to inform his father about his changing life plans, he continues. "Consequently, with great trepidation, I remember telling my father that, in my senior year I wanted to drop Air Force ROTC, where I was the aspiring Wing Commander, and enroll in all of the sciences courses to prepare for medical school. It would mean that I would have to spend an additional year beyond graduation to qualify. I told my father I didn't want to go into business with him. Anticipating a great storm, and much to my surprise, he said, 'That's wonderful.' In retrospect, I speculate he was thinking to himself, 'Oh wow, my son the doctor!' While Dad was successful business-wise, it would be quite something to have a physician in the family."

"I went back to Notre Dame, completed the necessary studies, and went on to medical school." Two years later, Lynn recalls a conversation with his father, who asked, 'Why did you change directions? You had a golden platter before you.' "I told him that I didn't like the politics involved in business. I knew that if you didn't play politics and give gifts at times to your customers, they might go elsewhere to do business. 'There is no politics like that in medicine,' I said. Then my dad started to chortle. He said, 'Son, there *are* politics in medicine.' I responded that it couldn't be as bad as business, which today of course, may be just the opposite."

> "No man can be responsible for another human being until he strives to be awakened in himself an inner force that can take responsibility for his own mental, emotional and physical impulses."
>
> —Jacob Needleman
> *The Way of the Physician*
> (1985)

After medical school, an internship, and a stint in the US Navy as a flight surgeon, Lynn completed a 4-year residency in urology. He then practiced as a board-certified urologist for 10 years. He eventually came to grips with his alcoholism. He realized that he suffered from the disease and started on the road to recovery. The experience stimulated him to consider becoming a care provider in this field as well as a receiver of care. He says, "There is in our field something we affectionately refer to as 'the savior syndrome.' I got a whiff of this and decided it was something I probably should explore. So I began pursuing addiction education by attending conferences."

According to Jim, while working with clients in career development over the years, it is not unusual for people to discover vocational passion as a consequence of a tragedy or illness. It may cause us to take a new road and discover that our key enjoyable skills are engaged by such a journey. Mothers Against Drunk Driving (MADD) is a visible example.

Lynn continues, "After some disc surgery, I went to Florida to recuperate. Whereupon, my wife, who often has more insight than I do, observed that urology didn't have the same passion for me as before. She asked if I ever thought about helping people with alcohol problems. After thinking and praying about it, we decided to engage in a new journey down this path. Without having a job, we decided to move to Florida. It seemed like the right thing to do and I had a sense of being led in this direction. I started studying to obtain a Florida medical license and we put our home in Illinois on the market."

"When I told my staff and colleagues about plans to move in a few months, they told me that I had lost my mind. But again, by coincidence and in a round about way, I had an opportunity to speak with a physician who knew of an addiction unit in Lakeland, Florida, that needed a medical director. I applied for the position and was accepted. After 2 years in this program, I was recruited to direct the largest hospital-based addiction treatment program in the state where I spent 9 years. It was at this time that I became enamored with specifically treating physicians and their special nuances."

"In 1992 I had coronary bypass surgery and it became apparent again that someone was attempting to get my attention and that I needed a lifestyle change." He recalls the scene, "I was standing in the shower, shaving the hair off my chest so they could perform the surgery the next day. My wife was afraid I was going to die, so she was not in a good emotional state. She walked into the bathroom and said, 'Some jerk doctor from the state of Washington is on the phone and wants to know if you want to run their physician health program. You wouldn't be interested in that, would you?' "I said, 'Of course not. That's the most ridiculous thing I ever heard of.' Then the light went on. After surgery, we packed for Seattle."

Working with chemically dependent physicians has become Lynn's passion. It is not simply addiction medicine, but working with physicians who are in trouble with chemicals and who have other kinds of health problems.

We asked whether chemical dependency is on the rise among physicians today. "I don't think it's on the rise, but the number of physicians we are reaching is on the rise. There are multiple reasons for this increase. First, we have done a tremendous job in educating the medical community about the fact that these doctors are not weak-willed or bad. They are sick. If you detect signs and symptoms early enough and get them into appropriate treatment, they enjoy tremendous success. Today there is a heightened awareness that doctors, as well as their patients, can become ill. They are human beings as well as human doers."

During his visits around the state, Lynn hears physicians saying that if there were a way out of medicine, they would leave the profession. He hears stories about investments in apple orchards and in numerous types of franchises. On a personal level, he reports, "My son, a Navy corpsman, had to decide during the past year whether to go to medical school or be a physician assistant. He chose the latter, primarily because of life style." This correlates with Jim's experience of working with younger people during career planning workshops. He administers a Career Anchors instrument that includes nine generic work values, one of which is called Lifestyle Balance. Approximately two thirds of participants completing the instrument list lifestyle balance as their first or second priority value.

We asked Lynn where he sends sick physicians to receive treatment. "We conduct an initial screening assessment, then we send them off for a multidisciplinary, comprehensive evaluation. We seem to be getting more complex cases these days. They will have chemical dependency as well as other mental illness issues. Unfortunately, these assessments require much time to complete. Physicians often are not easy to deal with, so we have to send them to places having experience in dealing with their nuances. Generally, physicians do not make good patients."

He amplifies, explaining, "For MDs, providing health care to patients and reaching out for it personally are almost mutually exclusive. For this reason, because of their special expertise, there are only a few places throughout the country with expertise in dealing with the doctor as patient."

We asked about local support groups for physicians, such as Caduceus groups. He answered by saying that the term "Caduceus group" is all inclusive. While it means different things in different places, these Caduceus groups are limited to serving health care professionals who are chemically dependent. "They take on different forms depending upon the locale," Lynn explains. "Some groups include only physicians, while other groups may include nurses, paramedics, counselors, and physical therapists. Some groups provide only mutual support, giving members the opportunity of discussing their recovery as it relates to their practices. Others take on the flavor of Alcoholics Anonymous, although not in an official sense because they restrict themselves to health care professionals. A group called the International Doctors in AA has more than 6,000 members." Lynn states that his program has its own groups totally separate from the others, although they encourage their clients to participate in AA.

In today's challenging environment, apart from getting help for a particular problem, we were curious about how physicians can take care of themselves physically, mentally, and spiritually. He says, "We are looking at how we can be more proactive in providing support groups for people affected by all the stress that is in the profession. We have a few groups operating in the Seattle area, and we are watching them closely to see if they should be replicated or modified. But, as I said earlier, [the idea of] doctors providing care to others and asking for help are almost mutually exclusive. In terms of physical concerns, MDs get lousy care. You won't get many positive responses if you go to any medical conference and ask for a show of hands of those physicians having had a physical examination in the past year. Few have their own personal physician."

"Participation in support groups by doctors who are not necessarily impaired could help immensely because they allow the individual to identify as being part of the greater whole," Lynn believes. "But, the problem is," he says, "though a commonality exists, if they are not professionally facilitated, they tend to turn into bitch sessions. When doctors participate for 3 or 4 weeks and don't see any improvement or bonding, they quit.

"Unfortunately," he says, "everything in their training mitigates against this kind of involvement. If you attend a wedding, you might see four doctors talking to each other in a corner. They are not interacting with the rest of the people because they never developed good interpersonal skills. They're in the library or the laboratory when everyone else is going out having pizza or going to a football game. It reinforces our isolation."

"We are not good at taking care of ourselves. We have difficulty in reaching out and admitting our humanity. As MDs, we have been deified for too long. First, we were told during medical school that you don't get sick. If you are sick, you better show up anyway. In addition, if we take any time off, an immediate guilt mechanism takes over." Lynn is convinced that if physicians are going to take care of themselves, it must involve a paradigm shift. "And," he emphasizes, "it will have to begin back in medical school where the word 'balance' gets inserted into the vocabulary. This is not an easy task. Some institutions around the country are looking at this. They will set aside a few days to take people on a retreat, focusing upon personal well-being. I hope that physicians just beginning to get into trouble would seek some professional assistance, but currently I have doubts about it."

Lynn's remarks caused us to reflect upon insights offered by Adolf Guggenbühl-Craig in his book, *Power in the Helping*

Professions. He writes about the physician archetype. Coined by Carl Jung, an archetype is not a static principle but an image residing within us that contains tremendous energy. Guggenbühl-Craig states, "In archetypal situations the individual perceives and acts in accordance with a basic schema inherent in himself [or herself]."[8] He asserts that to heal truly, the patient must participate in the process by engaging the power of this inner physician. In concrete terms, among other activities, this involves taking responsibility to follow the physician's advice and treatment.

The reverse is equally true. The physician has constellated in herself or himself a "patient archetype," resulting in the concept of the "wounded healer." If the "patient" psychologically residing within the physician is denied or repressed, the physician tends to deify himself or herself. "The doctor no longer is able to see his own personal wounds, his own potential for illness; he sees sickness only in the other." [9]

Admitting his frustration and feeling overwhelmed with providing reactive care through the Physician Health Program Lynn directs, he confesses, "We are putting out fires all the time in terms of dealing with disease. I would like to take a more preventive stance, but it's difficult to do with the available resources. Every 3 days we get a new phone call about some doctor who is in trouble. I would love to reach them before the difficulties begin. We are far from this possibility at the moment."

Since much of our conversation reflected his current work, we shifted subjects to ask about his understanding of the meaning of the word "soul." "Soul," Lynn believes, "is the core or essence of your total being, that underlying principle from which you derive your existence. It becomes a guiding light that hopefully will direct you to that path allowing you to self-actualize to the highest degree."

He sees a close relationship between soul and spirituality. "Spirit is very close to soul," he adds. "Spirit becomes a manifestation of the soul's work. You may not be able to see it, but you can feel spirit at work. It emanates from an individual or a group connected to soul. I would define spirituality as the condition

---

[8] Guggenbühl-Craig A. *Power in the Helping Professions.* Irving, TX: Spring Publications; 1979: 85.
[9] Guggenbühl-Craig A. *Power in the Helping Professions.* Irving, TX: Spring Publications; 1979: 94.

existing when an individual has a harmonious relationship with himself, his fellow human beings, and a power greater than himself." (The reader may note the connection between this statement and the music metaphor mentioned in the introduction to this book.)

From his perspective, we asked Lynn to describe a physician who is connected to soul and spirit. "First of all, he (she) would be enjoying life. He would be effervescent and excited about his endeavors. He would have things in perspective, wherein balance reigns. It would be someone who is very self-directed and self-rewarded. I would call such a person as being 'allocentric' as opposed to egocentric. It means not being caught up in oneself, not being self-centered, but being harmoniously connected in community with people and nature while maintaining a strong sense of personal identity."

For example, and in more concrete terms, we suggest that allocentric experiences frequently occur during the sharing and listening to life stories without judgment. The individual's identity is preserved and even expanded; yet often there is a deep sense of interconnectedness. Stories cojoin when we hear someone say, "I had a similar experience."

As with other physicians interviewed, we questioned Lynn about his optimism or pessimism for the future of health care in the United States. He says frankly, "I think it's going to get worse before it gets better. The one positive trend I see is physicians are finally realizing that they do have some clout, in contrast to several years ago when a group of doctors couldn't even agree about the time of the day." Emphatically, he adds, "We must be responsible for our own destiny and step up to the plate; I'm beginning to see this happening. We now realize we have been victims of 'divide and conquer' by all of the external forces, whether lawyers, accountants, or managed care officials. However, it will require some time for the medical community to gear up for the fight against these very powerful external powers. When that happens, I will become optimistic about the future."

"But, at the present time," he notes soberly, "we've lost what I call the three A's. We no longer have autonomy, ability, or authority to practice medicine. This is driving physicians away from medicine, and this must be restored. It's not just about money; that's part of the problem, but not the major issue. There were 103 students in my graduating class at medical school. We once took a straw vote, asking how many of us were in medicine for the money. Only one student raised his hand. At least he was honest, but the rest of us thought he was a jerk."

In summary, Lynn mentioned a phrase that prevails in the recovery field. "An old physician who treated a lot of alcoholics back in the late 60s and early 70s offered it. He spoke about the transformation of recovery, the entire psychological change occurring when someone recuperates. The saying is a joke about someone who is attempting to claim that he is in recovery. In a picture, he wears a button on his chest saying that he is in recovery, but the bottom of the picture reads 'We'll know it when we see it.' A similar saying in the medical field states that you can't give away something you don't have. You can't just talk the talk without walking the walk first. My biggest plea for the medical profession would be that you can't effectively function as a physician if you are not whole yourself. You can't pass it on because you haven't got it to give. This is the greatest threat to the profession. Therefore, my plea is to implement the kinds of changes that are necessary in medical schools and at the practice level that allow a physician to enrich his or her soul, and then to manifest that spirit in its entirety."

FAITH-BUOYED CAREGIVERS

"Gratitude is the parent of all other virtues."
—**Cicero**

RevDoc

Wayne Steven Martin, MD, MDiv

We sat in Dr Wayne Martin's small comfortable office surrounded by his collection of the biographies of early physicians, one of his passions. On the walls hang many first and early editions of stamps depicting medical themes. Proudly, he points out one of Albert Schweitzer. "One of my disappointments," he says, "is that I didn't get to Africa to meet him." Schweitzer is only one of Wayne's heroes; others include John Wesley and Sir William Osler.

Wayne's office is located in the oldest physicians' office structure in the small rural western Washington town where he lives. The original small house has been expanded and added on to over the years. Yet, it still maintains the atmosphere of a small-town family practice. A native of the community, Wayne's family, on both his paternal and maternal side, goes back more than 100 years. His dream to return to the Skagit Valley was fulfilled when he returned to open his medical practice.

Although he has been practicing family medicine since 1984, medicine is actually a second career. Growing up on a farm, Wayne always had a tender spot for others, whether animals or human beings. His parents also owned a meat-packing plant. He recalls, "I was involved in the daily butchering process. That's a kind of paradox, but that's how I began to learn about anatomy. I really did not enjoy slaughtering animals."

"Of course, at an early age, you dream of various kinds of occupations," he continues. "I thought I would enjoy being an engineer on a train. I still get a thrill when I see Amtrak going by," he grins. "My father served as a medic during World War II. He would meet the planes returning from bomb runs and treat those who were wounded or pick up the dead. He had a lot of innate medical skills. I can remember as a child the times he treated us when we were ill." Interestingly, today Wayne is his physician.

Wayne's first career choice was as a Methodist minister. Immediately following his undergraduate studies, he went to seminary, spending 4 years in school including a year overseas. After serving a parish in eastern Washington for 5 years, he changed career directions. Even though he felt comfortable with many aspects of being a pastor, he realized, as he put it, that medicine was an itch that needed scratching. And though he especially enjoyed counseling and working with young people, the call of doctoring remained strong in his psyche. Also, during his year in the Philippines as a seminary intern, he developed a significant feeling for mission work.

He declares, "I was there at a time when many of the pastoral duties were being turned over to the indigenous population. I wanted to return to mission work in the country, but knew I would have to return in a specialty different from pastoring. This reality was also part of the reason for exploring medicine."

When his first wife left him, it complicated his life as a minister, but freed him to consider a different vocation. However, at age 32 he found it impossible to be accepted into a US program, so he went to Mexico, spending 4 years in Guadalajara. "That was another experience," he relates, "because I didn't speak any Spanish when I arrived. The school provided a crash course, a requirement before matriculation. Myself and hundreds of other Americans were enrolled at that time."

When Wayne returned from Mexico, he took a fifth clinical year in Chicago, bringing him up to speed with other US graduates. He was 41 years old when he began his practice, older than any other person in the program. After practicing in Chicago for a few years, he decided to return to his home state.

Acceding to the call of medicine for Wayne was listening to his vocational passion. "Passion," according to Wayne, "implies a love of your work. You would perform it even if you were not paid, which sometimes seems to be on the brink of reality in the profession," he adds a little ruefully. His advice to his daughter as she graduates from high school is to find something to do with her work life that she will enjoy regardless of the money.

A good physician, notes Wayne, is one who offers affability, availability, and affordability to patients. "In my general practice, I don't see people paying much attention to educational background other than the fact that you've jumped through all the hoops," he states. "They want to know if you are available in case of an emergency in the middle of the night. In our clinic, we even make house calls. We don't make many, of course, but I will visit a few patients who cannot leave home. In addition, it really helps to experience their home environment. You can learn so much by seeing what life is like in a person's home. People are amazingly gracious when we visit them like this; they appreciate the extra effort."

Our homes often represent a safe, secure, and soulful place for us. In his book, *Sacred Space*, Clif Cleaveland, MD, speaks reverently of a painting by Samuel Luke Fildes, titled *The Doctor*. It depicts a physician in concerned contemplation visiting the home bedside of a sleeping or comatose child. The child's arm hangs slightly over the edge of a blanketed bed. Dr Cleaveland says, "Fildes [through this picture] defines a sacred space, or circle of caring, whose center is a terribly sick or injured fellow mortal."[1] While understanding the economic liabilities in today's health care environment, we suspect that such home visits heighten the experience of sacred space for Wayne and his associates.

Wayne also has a large reproduction of Fildes' painting on the wall of his office. Deeply moved by it, he gives it a slightly different twist, suggesting one interpretation might be that the child in the picture may be the physician's own child. Hence, the image is one of helpless concern on the part of the physician father.

Wayne considers his deep sense of wanting to help his patients as one of his key, nontechnical skills. He states, "We all have human limitations, including limitations of how illness and disease can be treated, so it's important not only to like, but sometimes actually love, patients." As he tells us, he always asks questions that go beyond physical concerns. "I don't think it's just idle chat; you want to how more about them so you can help them on a broader scale. I can get into some really deep discussions with my patients."

"Of course," he adds, "I don't wear my reverend title on my sleeve, although my license plate says 'Revdoc.' But, a lot of people know that I am a minister, and we will chat about subjects that are important to them, and sometimes about spiritual issues. At least 60% to 70% of the people I see have some spiritual issue affecting their health. In fact, that may be true of almost all of them. I certainly don't push such issues, but I have prayed with patients on an as-needed basis. I've really not had anyone who was opposed to prayer; most people like that."

"In fact, I've participated in several funerals. Either the patient or the family might request my involvement. In either case, I've attended a lot of them, something that many physicians will avoid.

---

[1] Cleaveland C. *Sacred Space*. Philadelphia, PA: American College of Physicians; 1998: xvii.

I've puzzled about that, and I know, myself, that sometimes you feel so overwhelmed about the possibility that we didn't do something to prevent the death. I know it may seem a little suspicious to some people. It's like, 'If I can't get you better, I'll do the funeral,'" he smiles. Tongue in cheek, Wayne calls it a package deal. However, some of his patients do not have a church connection and, during the process of dying, he has been present, not only in the capacity of a physician, but as a fellow traveler in life.

He continues, "I conducted the funeral of a colleague who had not been a patient of mine, but a fellow doctor and a mentor to me. I know it was deeply appreciated and served as part of my personal grief process. In addition, my second grade teacher was a patient of mine and passed away. I didn't conduct the service, but attended it and was able to speak about what she meant to me. It's been interesting to be a part of people's lives in this respect."

Wayne believes that knowing the stories of his patients and, in turn, their knowing something about his life story, contributes to the effectiveness of his practice. Of course, some of his patients are there for the specific treatment of a problem; they really don't want a relationship beyond these services. And, unfortunately he maintains, "Some of the insurance products foster this kind of impersonal arrangement. But that's not the way I desire to practice medicine and it is one of the reasons I moved back home to Washington."

"However, some people seek me out because they know I am a 'Christian' physician, and for some of them, it makes a difference." Obviously, it makes no difference in terms of technical expertise. "It's a fine balance," he notes. "I don't want to be a bleeding heart about what I have done or how I feel about it. But, many of my patients and I have shared intimate aspects of our lives."

Not long before we interviewed him, Wayne's partner experienced a massive heart attack. "I was gratified that people really cared about him and about me," he says. "They realized that things were pretty tough because we had a fine relationship and also, I had to treat many of his patients. But it's really nice when people inquire about how *you* are doing and how they might help out."

About 2½ years ago, Wayne broke his ankle. Because the early X rays didn't clearly reveal a break, he walked on it for 5 or 6 weeks before realizing that it was broken. Subsequently, his orthopedist had to perform three surgeries, and Wayne was on crutches for weeks on end.

"I'm still having difficulty," he says, "and I will probably need additional surgery. In the meantime, our clinic has been reduced from three to two doctors, meaning a lot of overtime for me. But, people are quite gracious in their concern and offer to help in any way possible. I feel good about being accepted as the wounded healer," he acknowledges. "When I was a minister, we used to say that we are dying men and women preaching to dying men and women. We are all on a continuum of health. Physicians are not immune to this stuff."

Working hard and doing double-time, as he puts it, is the kind of practice he sought. "If I had wanted a walk-in clinic or ER work, you wouldn't have the relationship," he says earnestly. "People call us up when we are not on call or on our way out of town. Our phone number is in the book; we don't hide. We're part of the community. That's the way we wanted it."

We asked Wayne what he would want people to say about him at the end of his life. He responds laughingly, "One of my more irritable patients told me that he overheard some women speaking about me, saying 'I hope he doctors better than he preached.' But I guess I would want people to say, 'Yes, he would get up in the middle of the night to see me, and that he did have a sense of humor about it.' I would also want them to say that my gifts and talents perhaps weren't perfect but that I did the best I could with what I had."

Like all physicians, Wayne isn't perfect. Being sensitive to doing his best by his patients, he acknowledges setbacks in his practice. "There have been a couple and these usually revolve around patients where I feel I haven't done my best. I think the most searing happened not long after I got back. I saw a fellow my age as a patient with whom I had played as a kid. He had multiple health conditions, some of which were caused by lifestyle and personal health decisions. He was only 45 years old when he died. There was little I could do for him, but I felt horrible. I was just devastated. Here was someone with whom I grew up who came to me and trusted me. I felt horribly that I hadn't done my best for this friend, this patient. I went to the funeral with a kind of soul sickness; it was just awful. His wife had been widowed before." Fearing that a medication change he prescribed might have contributed to his friend's death, even though the multiple medical conditions make the medication an unlikely factor, Wayne continues to think about the circumstances.

"I became really depressed. It knocked me for a loop," he confesses. "My wife and my daughter were aware of my suffering. I was able to share a lot of this with them, and I think that slowly with my background of faith I was able to pull out of it. I still think about it. I plumbed the depths of my soul and as a result I felt more resilient. Now I face situations better knowing I am not perfect."

Wayne does not deliver babies. "I haven't really done it since residency. That was by choice. When I was a senior resident I saw so many tragedies. I knew that would just simply unglue me. I really intended to do that before my graduation and I spent extra time so I could do my own C-sections. Although, if I ever return to mission work, that is certainly something I would have to do. I have also found getting closer to age 60 that is it harder to get up at night. Many physicians give up delivering babies close to this time of life." Much of Wayne's practice today is filled with geriatric patients.

Acknowledging that he is different today than when he started his practice, he laughs, "I hope I am. When I started, it was all so new and exciting. Years and experience have kind of tempered a lot of that. I don't like to use the words less idealistic, but probably my expectations and reality are little closer together. I still like to think I am idealistic. I enjoy reading about the lives of other physicians, how they ended up in medicine, and that inspires me along the way."

"I don't have a solo practice because I appreciate the camaraderie with others. With my partner out these last months, I am grateful for the opportunity of bouncing things off others. I appreciate the camaraderie at the hospital, seeing how they are doing and perhaps encouraging them on their journeys."

Prayer is an important component in his approach to medicine. "When I see a patient, I will pray before going into the room. I will pray that I will listen in the presence of Christ. I almost feel that something is happening—energy. I hear their [patients'] stories and more often come out feeling more healed than them. I almost feel that something is happening as I am listening to what they are saying. Often times, even if I had thought beforehand that this wasn't going to be a good experience, if I am intentional about what I am doing, and I don't mean that in a mechanistic sense, but in a caring, listening, empathetic way, then all kinds of good things can happen. I discover more and more it can be a therapeutic encounter for me."

Wayne believes the power to heal ultimately comes from God. He explains, "It can come in many different ways." According to Wayne, one way this may occur is through using our intellect and minds to develop new antibiotics and new ways of treating diseases.

"As much as I have studied theology and medicine, I am still surprised by the healing process and the variations and aspects of it. Often it comes through our skills. I think it reflects the love that is universal to God. There is spontaneous healing, but I think that is pretty rare. I think God can and probably does work in some ways that you might classify as miracles. But, I think also that our skills and our ability to lean into the healing process and get in line with that power is probably where most of the healing comes."

With the ongoing changes in medicine, Wayne remains hopeful. "What makes me hopeful about medicine is thinking about all the people who are willing to make the sacrifice to go into medicine to help people. They may receive less remuneration and experience greater stress, but I believe in the basic patient–doctor relationship."

Intrinsic Soul Healer

Joy Kim, MD

"I consider myself a soul healer," Joy Kim says, smiling, eyes twinkling as she leans forward earnestly. Joy's bubbling enthusiasm for her faith serves as the underpinning of her work as a family practice physician. And, while she speaks freely using distinctively religious terminology, at no time did we hear her using exclusive language. She honors all faith systems and never attempts to proselytize.

While listening to Joy, we reflected upon how people often journey through periods of transition successfully and mature as individuals. The map is not the territory; but like all symbols or representations of ultimate reality, models have been formulated describing the stages or phases of faith development. Not unlike Maslow's hierarchy of needs, the phases begin with elemental concerns and progress toward maturation.

Of course, trust in and of itself is a basic necessity. Without a basic sense of trust, we could not survive. A child must trust in parents or in someone to meet basic needs of food, warmth, and security. Here, hopefully the foundation is laid to progress through adolescence to adulthood.

In a similar manner, James Fowler [2] and others have formulated phases of faith development. We describe them very briefly:

- Level One represents the *forming* stage, where the basic "rules" of faith are fashioned in terms of right and wrong. Generally, moral issues are black or white. Here, great importance is given to external authority, such as a person or a sacred scripture.

- Level Two describes a "we" kind of *conforming* to a community such as "we Presbyterians." It often includes conventional thinking and dependence on others.

- Level Three portrays a kind of adolescent rebellion or *storming* orientation, when authority is called into question and independent thinking flourishes.

---

[2] Fowler J. *Stages of Faith*. San Francisco, CA: Harper San Francisco; 1995.

- Level Four is often called the stage of *reforming* and integration. One's faith includes accepting and embracing paradox, to live with the sometimes frightening unknown.
- Finally, in Level Five we reach *transforming* time, realizing a sense of cohesion with God (or Being) and the universal community, as well as kind of self-transcendence.[3]

Joy's story reflects the kind of cohesion, community, and self-transcendence described in Level Five. For her, soul is where God comes to reside in us. She states, "It is the instrument that God created allowing us to have a relationship with Him. Soul will never die. Sometimes we see people who have a kind of deadened spirit, but the soul lives on, even when the body dies. It is a very special and precious place because, even though my thoughts and feelings are sometimes focused elsewhere, I know that my soul is still present."

Building on the work of psychologist Gordon Allport, in his book, *The Healing Power of Faith: Science Explores Medicine's Last Great Frontier*, Harold Koenig, MD, distinguishes between intrinsic and extrinsic faith systems. *Extrinsic* believers use religion to achieve their own purposes, such as finding friends or gaining status and power. They can be rigid at times and pass judgment on themselves and others. Many people are turned off or wounded by such extrinsic behaviors. In contrast, we experienced Joy's faith as intrinsic.

Intrinsic believers see faith as the central, motivating force in their lives. Feeling loved by God and empowered by this faith, their care giving is not motivated by personal gain. It is freely given in response to a gift. For those who may be uncomfortable with this kind of language, Koenig asserts,

> "Even if you lack strong faith, you might gain considerable health benefits by observing devoutly religious people and adopting some of their practices, perhaps community volunteer work."[4]

In the introduction to this book, we spoke of two worldviews. The one is of a world operating like a machine. The second is based on theoretical physics, viewing the world more like a living web. Joy especially embraces the second perspective.

---

[3] Barnhouse R. Mentioned in the Introduction, describes an agnostic as someone who is in between phases.

[4] Koenig H. *The Healing Power of Faith*. New York, NY: Simon & Schuster; 1999: 25.

"I don't think anything happens accidentally. In synchronicity, somehow everything mysteriously connects, whether we are conscious of it or not. What happens to me occurs for a reason, and God orchestrates it. Sometimes, of course, bad things happen to people, but I always think about what such an event teaches me. I view it as an incredible privilege to be in a place where I can see a lot of things coming together. That is why being a doctor is so awesome. Even little events and relationships harvest value during the course of a day or a year. For example, perhaps 5 years ago I cared for a patient, then suddenly today, I am helping this person again but in a different way. I sometimes ask myself about the significance of my actions. But then, later it begins to make sense." Several patients have told Joy that she was an answer to their prayer.

As Joy spoke about this mysterious connection, a poem came to mind, written by Lawrence Kushner in his book, *Honey From the Rock.* He asserts that everyone is born with one or several pieces of a puzzle and we never know how they might fit into another person's life. "And when you present your piece . . . to another, whether you know it or not, whether they know it or not, you are a messenger from the Most High."[5] Joy affirms, "You have a choice to use your piece of the puzzle or not. There are times when we get the prompting, and it is very difficult to pay attention unless you open up your spirit. When the only focus is on your personal agenda, you may miss an opportunity to affect healing in a more comprehensive manner."

When Joy was about 4 years old, she visited her aunt in Korea, where she was born and raised for a time. "My aunt was a family physician who lived in a very poor, industrial area. When I witnessed what she was doing, I knew that I wanted to follow in her footsteps," she remembers. Shrugging, she asks rhetorically, "Looking back, how does a 4-year-old know what she wants to do vocationally? So I perceive my practice as a calling. Of course, there were some periods in my life when I had doubts about the profession," she admits.

"After my mother's death during my adolescent years, I had reservations in terms of the time and energy involved in becoming a doctor. I knew at that time it was not going to be easy.

---

[5] Kushner L. *Honey From the Rock.* Woodstock, VT: Jewish Lights Publishing; 1990: 69–70.

I thought about what else I could do. But after a year of pondering over it, I decided that medicine was for me. At age 13, I began setting some goals. I became a candy striper and at age 17, I entered training to become a nurse's assistant. I decided on being an MD rather than a nurse because I was drawn to its greater challenge and higher accountability."

As a graduate student in the United States, Joy's father fell in love with its culture. Joy remembers her father promising to bring his family to America after having time to experience their Korean culture. "I was the youngest child, so he waited until my oldest brother was ready for college and I turned 10 before moving."

Joy speaks about moving around quite a bit during this period. In 1970, they left Korea and visited Los Angeles. Her father didn't like that environment, so they decided to move to Sao Paulo, Brazil. Due to what they believed to be a faulty education system, the family moved back to the United States, settling in Kansas City.

Joy's experiences as a young, Korean, female medical student contradict some people's perception that medical education is more difficult for women. "In medical school, I was treated very fairly. My cultural background was not a problem because, as you know, there is a lot of diversity."

She believes that it was easy and natural because she is in family practice, which has the potential for being very nurturing. "I didn't see it as overly masculine," she says. "Being a woman, it was quite easy to solicit a social as well as a medical history. I got to know people very well and easily connected with them. However, being of Asian background in a Caucasian community, I had some concerns to overcome. When beginning my practice in 1990, people would call and ask whether I spoke English very well or where I went to medical school. They also wanted to know how long I had been in this country," she laughs.

Medicine is definitely a passion for Joy, and it serves as her creative outlet. "But, to be honest, there were times in my life when I was very performance oriented," she admits. "Because I was Asian, I thought that I had to work harder than others. No one pressured me, but I pressured myself. Because of this, pride was a big issue. So when I began my practice, it was very conventional. That was when I lost some of the passion for medicine. I started the practice with a partner, feeling a huge obligation to succeed. I felt very burned out after about 4 years."

"Then, something shifted inside me." She confides, "My patients weren't responding to treatment as well as I wanted. Sometimes it is very difficult to get people committed to a diet or to stop smoking. Then I stumbled onto faith and spirituality. I had come from a Christian background, but earlier had no genuine relationship with Christ. After my mother died, I practically walked away from my faith. I attended church and some Bible studies, but I didn't know how to integrate this into my life. Burnout caused me to begin searching for meaning in my life. That's when I really met Jesus in a very intimate way. It suddenly came to me that I was loved and all I really had to do was love in return," she says and smiles. "I came to grips with emotional resilience. Even with a family, I didn't have to take on the burdens of life by myself."

"I firmly believe that we are on the brink of a great new era in medicine: a time when health professions will begin to help people regain control over their lives by providing them with the spiritual tools to maintain health and wellness."

— Harold Koenig, MD
The Healing Power of Faith
(1999)

"Today I teach that which I am learning myself. I like to teach people about what is working for me and what causes me to struggle," she tells us enthusiastically. "This is my passion, the journey I embraced 5 years ago."

"You could say I have regained the original passion I had for medicine. Some of the training robs you of that passion. Some of the things you must do in medical school and during residencies take away the 'get to' and replaces it with the 'have to.' It's a movement from 'You mean, I get to do this every day and get paid?' to 'I must make the grade.' It takes the joy out of medicine."

"Today I am more of a wounded healer. By learning about what this concretely means, I can offer so much more to people. I see myself as a wounded person being healed by God. My goal includes not only healing the body, but the soul as well."

Joy continues, "When I see a patient, it is usually because something is wrong physically. Sometimes the solution is quite simple, as with an infection. You prescribe an antibiotic and the infection goes away. In other situations, patients see me because of a chronic condition, something that reoccurs. Then healing may involve going beyond the symptom and exploring the root cause of it. Without putting blame on a person, I sometimes ask, what is this illness telling you? It includes asking God, our healer, to participate in the problem and in its solution. So the healing process steps beyond the symptoms, while putting compassion into the equation."

Joy's obvious integration of faith and spirituality into her medical practice prompted us to ask her to describe the characteristics of a physician who is considered a spiritual medical practitioner.

She responds thoughtfully, "I would say it is a doctor who explores beyond the physical symptoms. Whether using the word or not, everyone possesses a spirit, so for me a good doctor invests time and energy beyond the physical realm. It involves making a connection beyond just writing a prescription. A lot of us tend to want to 'fix things.' But some things can't be fixed by human efforts. All healing comes from God, our healer. So it includes connecting with one's personal spirit to see how it connects with another person's spirit. Obviously, it is difficult, if not almost impossible, to do this in a 5- to 10- minute office visit, although it can be done, which is what our culture has come to in patient care."

Using an example of a colleague, she continues, "Tom Cornwell [whose story is included in this section] comes to mind as a doctor who is very perceptive as he makes house calls. He visits a patient's home, as opposed to having them come to a sterile environment. He recognizes specific symbols and pictures displayed in a home and he solicits stories about them. So, he is involved in their whole being. I also think of an orthopedic doctor who looks not only at a bone, but goes well beyond it."

Joy connects with her patients spiritually whether or not they are aware of that fact. First, she informs us that she prays for almost every one of her patients, even though they may not know about it. She might not include in her prayers patients who simply come in for a physical, but she especially focuses on more difficult situations of patients who are generally not following her medical advice. She is adamant in her belief in the power of intercessory prayer. "There are books about this, but I did it even before I knew they were published. I am a very 'right-brain' person, so it comes naturally for me," she smiles.

"As a family doctor, I see a lot of people who have what I call a 'sad spirit.' They may be dealing with depression and relational issues. Therefore, when I pray for them, I simply ask what I am suppose to do for them. What am I to say? Sometimes I'll end up saying something that seems fairly wild, but what my patient needs to hear. Other times I will move into extended history taking that may include asking people about their spiritual history. If someone asks why I am probing them about this issue, I will simply quote a study showing the relationship between health and spirituality. It doesn't matter whether these people are Muslim, Jewish, or Christian, but it allows me to connect to their spirit and know where they are coming from. I'm not preaching to them. They may not share my perception of God. Obviously, if I see them wearing a cross or rosary, I'll comment that we have something in common and ask, 'Have you tried prayer? . . . because studies have shown. . . .'"

"For where there is love of man, there is also love of the art. For some patients, though conscious that their position is perilous, recover their health simply through their contentment with the physician."

— Hippocrates

Because of such experiences, Joy organized what she calls a "healing circle." She believes that many people are spiritually broken and don't understand the body/mind connection to healing. She attempts to provide her patients with an environment where they learn all of the different modalities of healing.

"We have a healing circle of people who meet every Thursday evening for 2 hours. There is no cost involved because I view it as a service and a gift that I want to give my patients. Today, some of my patients are bringing their friends. More than anything, I show the connection of body/mind/spirit to healing. It involves coming to understand the invisible and how it impacts that which we can see and touch. Again, I believe providing this service is part of my calling."

Describing the healing circle's process, she explains, "Often we begin the session with a period of sharing. Then participants are introduced to a number of tools and techniques, such as deep breathing. We also discuss the spiritual modalities. My ultimate purpose is to help them connect with their faith, which is a very important part of building emotional resilience. People who have a deep faith system have been shown to be healthier."

Joy compares the trust patients give to their physician who prescribes medication to the trust given to the spiritual dimension. As she says, in her experience, the patient hardly ever asks whether a medication is safe. He or she has inherent trust that the doctor is competent and that the medication will do no harm. "That's faith!" she tells them. "'You put faith in me. Now I want you to put faith in something larger.' I want people to revive hope. Faith is like a muscle. If you don't use it, it becomes atrophied."

Joy eagerly shares the healing circle's impact on the lives of some of the participants. "One lady with a master's degree in teaching, with her husband and children, moved to our area, and she lost the ability to function. She had many phobias and had several physical problems. She visited me out of desperation, and we began to treat her with some medication. We attempted to look beyond her symptoms in search for the root of the problems. During circle sessions, the group embraced her with compassion. Soon new relationships began to develop for her. She began to serve as a mentor to some of the others. A big step in our life came when she mustered the courage to take a trip overseas."

Remembering another story, Joy continues, "Another lady told me that she could not come to the healing circle because she was ashamed of her weight. However, one evening she appeared and shortly thereafter shared her embarrassment, which contributed to the release of her shame. Then other issues surfaced relative to her health and her marriage. After a few weeks of group partici-pation, she decided to open each day with self-affirmations, mak-ing choices about her lifestyle. The healing circle provided a life-line to climb out of the well of her depression. She enlisted the help of a Christian marriage counselor and began to see that she was using her weight as an excuse to blame herself for her rela-tionship problems."

"As part of the group process, I also engaged them in a 6-week series of self-discovery. We used several instruments and exercises to help expand individual identity. For example, we used the Keirsey version of the Myers-Briggs Type Indicator®.[6] It's all very positive, because many people spend much of their time focusing on negative aspects of themselves."

Although Joy embraces the spiritual, she admits that discussing such issues with her physician colleagues is hard. "It's difficult, because doctors are often so isolated. I believe this is why physi-cians can become burdened so easily. We live in individualized boxes. Some of my associates are aware of what I do, but I'm not sure whether they are interested beyond the surface." She is

---

[6] More information available at http://www.keirsey.com.

grateful for the considerable support from the midwestern hospital where she is on staff.

Joy remains optimistic about the current health care environment. "On a day-to-day basis, sometimes I can be quite pessimistic." Grinning, she confesses, "But I am a hopeful person by nature. For me, optimism is a gift. I attempt to focus on issues over which I have some control. I try to focus my energy and live in the moment. I also love challenges, so if a situation appears to be impossible, I often view it as an opportunity to learn and grow, remembering Philippians 4:13: "I can do all things through Jesus who gives me the strength." Besides, I have the power of my faith supporting me. I am so privileged to be God's instrument."

As Lawrence Kushner reminds us in his book, *Money From The Rock*,[7] no one has all the pieces to the puzzle of life, but Joy appears to have more than a few of them, mutually receiving her many talents and sharing them with others. We also suspect that her first name is no accident.

---

[7] Kushner L. *Money From The Rock*. Woodstock, VT: Jewish Lights Publishing; 1990.

Faithful Servant

E. Wayne Day, MD

In writing her book, *Losing Your Job—Reclaiming Your Soul*, Mary Lynn Pulley interviewed dozens of people who successfully transitioned through the trauma of job loss. She found them embracing three fundamental qualities that allowed them to move successfully to a new job or career. First, they possessed the quality of *resilience*, the ability to spring back from a setback and to learn from the experience, altering key assumptions about work and about themselves as the external environment changed. Second, over time, they had the ability to establish and participate in a *community* of support that provided encouragement during the darker days of their transitions. In addition, they engaged a *faith* system, allowing them to move forward even when the final destination remained unclear. By faith, Pulley refers not just to their adhering to a set of religious beliefs, but they "took responsibility for acting on their own behalf while trusting in something larger."[8]

In our opinion, Dr E. Wayne Day embodies all three of these qualities. His identity as a person is not seated exclusively in practicing medicine. As he says, "I can define myself beyond the role of the physician. The day will probably come when I will no longer practice medicine, but there are many other things I can do." This does not imply a lack of passion for his profession. Rather, his commitment to medicine is undergirded by his Christian faith.

In reflecting upon our visit with Wayne, we were drawn to the comments of Daniel Sulmasy, in his book *The Healer's Calling:*

> "All the elements that Jesus had at his disposal are at the disposal of health care professionals today as well. . . . No matter how sophisticated the technology of healing gets, true healing will involve these three very simple human elements: compassion, touch, and conversation."[9]

As a gynecologist practicing in a rural Northwestern community, Wayne engages each of these elements as he serves his patients.

---

[8] Pulley ML. *Losing Your Job—Reclaiming Your Soul*. San Francisco, CA: Jossey-Bass; 1997: 154.

[9] Sulmasy DP. *The Healer's Calling*. Mahwah, NJ: Paulist Press; 1997: 17.

To this day, he can't remember a particular time or event leading to his decision to choose medicine as a career. "I came from a very humble background and no one in my family worked in a degreed profession. When I was a boy, I wanted to be a pilot, but there was no particular strong motivation behind that idea. It was just one of those things that little boys talk about, like being a cowboy or fire-fighter. The first inkling that medicine might be a career occurred when I came back from Vietnam and enrolled in college. I was encouraged to become a doctor by one of my professors." He recalls, "I just thought to myself, 'OK, I'll try it.' I am a goal-oriented person, so I set myself an objective to move in this direction."

Wayne's interest in becoming an obstetrician and gynecologist evolved over time. His training exposed him to a variety of specialties in his third year of medical school where he especially enjoyed surgery. Internal medicine also interested him. Soon, he discovered that being an OB-GYN provided him with best of both worlds in that pregnant women often have other medical concerns needing to be addressed. The specialty also offered the opportunity of using his surgical skills. In addition, Wayne believes that women are easier to work with than men and thus are more likely to adhere to medical advice.

In contrast to some physicians' experiences, Wayne did not find medical school particularly abusive. On the other hand, he does admit, "Anyone who goes through medical school experiences some abuse. It's almost a kind of rite of passage. I look at it as being a part of the profession. Also, in medical school you are faced with the first time of cutting into up a cadaver, which introduces you to some psychological trauma. And, you are exposed to cutting into a live human being for the first time, or facing a person who is dying or who has died."

As did a number of other physicians interviewed, Wayne believes that medical schools need to provide more training to prepare students for dealing with the emotions of such moments, as well as helping to prepare young physicians to address the spiritual dimension of medicine.

In practice since 1979, Wayne makes a distinction between passion and compassion. He believes *compassion* implies an attitude toward a person or a group of people; *passion,* especially when used to describe one's vocation, reflects an individual feeling. But, he hesitates to describe his practice of medicine as his sole passion. Regretfully, he says, "It's not like it used to be.

Passion encompasses enthusiasm and energy. I believe that most physicians who have been in practice for a while find their enthusiasm blunted and their energy diminished. This stems from the medical climate emerging over the past several years. In particular, because of managed care and other developments, medicine has been forced into an environment harmful to quality patient treatment."

He believes that this climate pressures more and more physicians to view their practices primarily as a business rather than a healing art with a focus on the patient. "Today," he emphasizes, "too much attention is given to marketing, to how many patients you can see in a given day, and to the bottom line. Physicians agonize about maximizing investment in order to keep the doors open. Of course, the healing art of medicine remains as a major concern, but the shift has been away from the patient."

Given these comments, we asked Wayne whether he was optimistic or pessimistic about the future of medicine.

"I'm pessimistic," he confesses. "The only thing that may impact the current trend is if physicians can extract themselves from being torn between the patient and the insurance company. I came into practice toward the end of the golden era and into a time when we are deeply involved in insurance issues. The golden era reflected a period when doctors took care of patients, billed them, and let the patients maintain direct contact with the insurance company. However, during the past few decades, physicians, desiring to provide extra assistance with the paperwork, have placed themselves between the patient and the insurance provider. Because they control the funds, today these organizations exercise unholy power, putting undue pressure on physicians. Insurance companies make decisions for the patient and the physician based on economics. It becomes a daily grind to hassle with these companies on whether a person is going to be covered."

Some of the physicians interviewed for this book share the belief that the pendulum may shift again, especially if the public

"Medicine is hazardous duty with increasingly less combat pay. The people controlling the dollars are demanding shared risk, but at the same time they have no clue the risks we bear as physicians."

— Joseph Cramer, MD
Association Home Page
Utah Medical Bulletin (2000)

airs its disenchantment. Wayne disagrees and questions whether the government and the insurance companies would be willing to relinquish their power. He believes that a form of freedom may occur for wealthier people who have the ability to pay more for their medical needs, but thinks that the average person has no such luxury. In fact, he believes the situation may deteriorate to the point of rationing care because there are certain things the government will not fund. Hearing his concerns, we asked Wayne about his hope for his personal practice.

"I have none. For a number of reasons, I have already stopped doing obstetrics, and I think this is a trend for an increasing number of doctors. Traditionally, OB-GYN physicians remained in medicine well into their 60's. During the last 5 to 10 years of the practice, usually they focused more on gynecology. Today we see a shift in terms of doctors not only leaving OB earlier, but exiting medicine altogether. I got out of OB when I was just over the age of 50."

"In addition, unlike many others, so far I have managed to avoid signing any managed care contracts. I like to view this as an ongoing experiment in survival tactics." Smiling, he asks, "Will I be the little doctor who fought the good fight and won, or will managed care eventually cause me to end my practice?" More soberly, he continues, "Right now, managed care is winning. I see my practice gradually diminishing in numbers of patients to the point where it will cause a forced retirement."

His obvious frustration raised doubts in our mind as to how resilient he might be in times of transition. We asked Wayne if retirement were to come prematurely, what he would do with his life and his many talents? How does one connect with soul in the midst of such dismay? We found the answers in his deep commitment to his Christian faith.

He lights up in talking about his faith. "Right now I am already refocusing my energy by engaging in medical mission activities. I have already been on several trips and will be leaving on another excursion in a few months. I've been to Romania, Mongolia, China, and India. In October, my wife and I will be leaving for Kazakhstan. These are short-term medical mission trips, usually 3 weeks in duration, organized by various Christian organizations that already have people in the field and who act as liaisons. There are opportunities for longer visits. Later I may have the freedom to take them, but it is impossible for me to do so today because I still have a practice." And, he confesses that if he weren't practicing medicine, he might be playing the guitar, still in Christian ministry.

Wayne explained more about these trips and the numbers of people involved. "It depends on the needs of the missionary," he tells us. "You never know what you are getting into until you arrive on location. You may go in with the idea of doing surgery, but end up conducting lectures. It also depends on the focus of the trip and on immediate needs. Some trips are very evangelical. For example, the trip to India included the largest short-term medical trip ever to be organized. We had a group of 165 people, including physicians and support staff. I have also been on trips with as few as four people. This occurred in China, where we conducted clinics for the poor as well as lectured to local physicians. We went out into the smaller areas of the country where the missionaries where attempting to make some headway."

Returning to a discussion of his current practice, we asked Wayne about his thoughts on what makes a good physician.

"A good physician must have compassion, viewing a patient as more than someone with a medical problem. I hesitate using the term 'holistic' because it has a wide range of connotations these days, but a good doctor approaches the patient from a physical, mental, and spiritual viewpoint," he states. "When I went to medical school, the spiritual aspect was not discussed and the mental, dimension was given minimal attention."

When we asked him to identify the nonclinical skills that he brings to his patients, he said, "It would be better to ask my patients that question. It is difficult to be objective about oneself. But, I think I give my patients a sense of being at ease. Of course, in the context of an intimate GYN exam in which there is considerable touching, you must be extremely careful in your demeanor. It must always be professional but, on the other hand, in my specialty, it is very important to put women at ease. I don't want to be seen as acting one way in the office and in another way on the street."

Keeping congruent in who he is personally and professionally is important to him. "In the last few years," Wayne adds, "My staff and I have opened up our office to really minister to patients in an inclusive manner. For example, if a patient asks for a prayer, my staff can respond without coming to me for permission. We find this to be very effective ministry as well as medicine. Prayer and spirituality play a very important role in the healing process. Our patients know where we are coming from, if not directly, then at least by the music played in the office, which is distinctively Christian in nature. This opens the door for a more spiritual involvement. I have patients who request prayer prior to surgery. When I was doing OB, on the way home I always prayed for a baby that I had just delivered."

Wayne believes that the way he practices medicine is not very different today than when he began. "I have not changed in terms of how I practice medicine. I have not allowed interventions from insurance companies to dictate my actions. My philosophy has always been that I will not make decisions for patients, but my role is to provide education, and then let them make the decisions. One of the reasons why I did not go into managed care was that I didn't want others to narrow the patient's options."

All physicians have setbacks of one kind or another and Wayne certainly is no exception. "Malpractice is the ugly word, and I have been sued," he admits. "I think the statistics will show that every obstetrician will be sued between three to five times during his career. Often, we think of ourselves as professionals being invincible to this, believing that if we take good care of people we will never be sued. That's putting your head in the sand. But when you are served with your first lawsuit, you tend to take it very personally. To an extent, it tends to be a setback in terms of one's level of confidence."

> "You cannot hope, of course, to escape from the cares and anxieties incident to the professional life. Stand up bravely, even against the worst."
>
> — Sir William Osler, MD
> *Aequanimitas* (1932)

However, he is quick to add, "You grow from this by not becoming cynical and by not falling into the trap of 'It's me against them.' You don't become defensive and begin ordering a lot of unnecessary tests and procedures. We all make mistakes, but fortunately I haven't made any of a very serious nature, such as the death of a patient. When I make a mistake in a diagnosis and in treatment, I attempt to be honest with people. If there is a problem, I visit with them and discuss the treatment, what may have gone wrong, and what could have been done in a better way. Then the patient decides what to do about the situation. My experience is that honesty is the best policy, and unless there has been major damage, people are willing to forgive."

Most of the physicians with whom we spoke talked about the wonder and mystery they experience in their practice. Wayne was no different and readily spoke about such experiences with enthusiasm. "That's easy to answer; childbirth stands out. Unfortunately, I had to give this up. But I continue to experience this wonderment, especially in terms of being a medical missionary. The arena has simply shifted."

We asked whether Wayne's sense of spirituality has changed over the years. "My relationship with the Lord has definitely deepened, but I don't think that has generally come about because of medicine. The spiritual focus of my wife and me has been more outside the medical community. We have other activities, particularly within our church. However, this deepening of spirituality has been very helpful in terms of medicine."

Not surprisingly, Wayne's primary hero is Jesus Christ. "This would be true of any Christian; he is the guiding light and the standard. I may not do a very good job of living up to this standard, and I think this is an issue in Christianity. Too many non-Christians look at us as being hypocritical and being untrue to the faith. But, like everyone else, we fall short of the mark." Wayne's thoughts echo why the earliest Christians were called "People of the Way," not having arrived yet at the final destination.

The importance Wayne places on personal integrity and honesty are reflected in two of his other heroes. Referring to Harry Truman, he says, "He was a person who stood by his guns and even though he may not have been a shining example of a Christian, at least he was honest and made difficult decisions even when it wasn't popular." Wayne adds, "Sam Nunn was another hero of mine. He was always a person who I thought had integrity and who demonstrated it in the Senate."

Wayne's deep personal beliefs also define his understanding of healing, believing that the power to heal "resides with the Lord." He explains, "I see the practice of medicine as a God-given gift. We are fortunate and carry within us a deep sense of responsibility, but there is a lot more healing involved than in what we can do with a knife or with medication. Physicians can impact patients and families beyond simply treating their illnesses. I think this is what a lot of patients desire. The problem we face today revolves around time issues, especially if someone is restrained by managed care."

"Because of time constraints and other issues, I know of some doctors who have walked away from medicine entirely, closing the door and turning in their licenses. That is a shame," he says sadly, "because there are so many opportunities, if not in the US, then in other areas of the world. You can make a difference."

Projecting into the future, we wonder what Wayne hopes people will say about him as a physician and a person. "Again, it relates to spirituality," he says. "Probably the best thing they could say is that he took care of me beyond my physical needs, and that he was a friend as well as a doctor."

His favorite poem, *Footprints in the Sand*, reflects his thoughts:

Last night I had a dream. I dreamed I was walking along the beach with the Lord. Across the sky flashed scenes from my life. For each scene, I noticed two sets of footprints in the sand: one belonged to me, the other to the Lord.

After the last scene of my life flashed before me, I looked back at the footprints in the sand. I noticed that at many times along the path of my life, especially at the very lowest and saddest times, there was only one set of footprints.

This really troubled me, so I asked the Lord about it. "Lord, you said once I decided to follow you, You'd walk with me all the way. But I noticed that during the saddest and most troublesome times of my life, there was only one set of footprints. I don't understand why, when I needed You the most, You would leave me."

The Lord replied, "My son, my precious child, I love you and I would never leave you. During your times of suffering, when you could see only one set of footprints, it was then that I carried you."

Author Unknown

Medicine as Gift

Martin C. Doot, MD

Medicine is more than a passion for Dr Martin Doot; it is a gift. As he tells us, "Passion, as defined by *Webster's Collegiate Thesaurus*, is an 'intense, high-wrought emotion that compels us to action.' I believe God gives us particular gifts and personalities that uniquely equip us for having purpose on earth. Specifically, we carry, realized or not, with a certain yearning to make a difference in a particular area—a passion for an explicit human need. As Frederick Buechner writes, 'Your vocation (calling) is to be found where your deep joy meets the world's deep need.'"

> "All physicians look for more meaningful lives than we realize. Being human is not unprofessional. Meaning is a function of the heart."
>
> — Rachel Naomi Remen, MD
> *Kitchen Table Wisdom* (1996)

Martin offers his experience of entering medicine as evidence of it being a gift. "I came to medicine in the same way I was led to my personal faith," he recounts. "My father wasn't a doctor, but a hard-working guy who didn't have the opportunity to go to college. He was a professional photographer. I think he was disappointed he didn't get the chance to use his intelligence in a way that was more useful. So, when I was a little kid starting to talk about being a doctor, at times he wanted it more than me. It caused real struggles between us, because when I began expanding my interests elsewhere, he tended to pull me back so I wouldn't fail in my schooling and my goals for medicine. He also introduced me to my faith, his faith becoming my faith and my goals becoming his goals for me."

While attending a Christian college for 2 years, Martin met his future wife. His four semesters of philosophy framed his thoughts and prepared him for scientific studies. "Our professor, Dr Calvin Seerveldt, taught us that everyone begins with some faith foundation and there is no need to apologize for it. He gave me strong academic confidence in my personal faith before getting into the rigors of the scientific field. Throughout my entire career, science never caused me to doubt that faith. I just accepted that science would teach me one dimension of my vocation."

He then enrolled at the University of Illinois to finish his undergraduate degree. Through his association with the

Intervarsity Christian Fellowship, Martin began a Bible study in his house, inviting his Jewish and Catholic roommates, among others, to take part. Martin realized they participated out of curiosity about the source of his faith. During this time, he struggled with whether to pursue medicine or ministry. One experience with another Catholic roommate had a profound impact on Martin's career direction.

"We spoke about faith, spirituality, and our goals in life," Martin states. However, he was more interested in experiences with hallucinogens than spirituality. Then, one day I came home from school, and he was crying. His mother had a heart attack. Not feeling adequate, he asked me to pray for her. This experience caused me to integrate my faith and my desire to be a doctor. I remember clearly thinking I would have an opportunity to share my faith during times of medical crises. Right then, I made a commitment to enter medicine and to carry my faith with me into my work."

However, getting to medical school proved to be a challenge. Martin clearly remembers his frustration over being rejected after applying to several medical schools. "Spring vacation arrived during my senior year, but no letter of acceptance came from any school. My fiancé trained to be an elementary teacher, but she didn't have a job. So, our futures were totally up for grabs. Discouraged, during spring break, I went to Loyola School of Medicine. A wonderful secretary in the admission's office looked at my file and said, 'I don't know why they haven't interviewed you. I'll rub it under their noses for you,'" he says laughing at the recollection. While visiting his fiancé out of town, he got a call from his father saying Loyola wanted to interview him. As he was leaving her apartment, his fiancé received a phone call from the administrator of a Christian school in Cicero, three suburbs east of Loyola, offering her a teaching position.

Three Loyola staff physicians interviewed Martin. At the end of his campus visit, he was informed that the dean wanted to see him again. "I can still picture his face," he says laughing. "Dean Rich was a psychiatrist who, with his full beard, looked the part. He said, 'I spoke to two of the physicians who interviewed you. We have decided you are a very acceptable candidate for our medical school. You're in!'"

"With tears in my eyes, I walked out into the parking lot and thanked God. My vision of becoming a doctor and integrating

spirituality with medicine began to unfold. I considered it a gift
and not something that I earned."

Throughout his clinical rotations, no specialty particularly
interested him. Finally, because it was something essentially different from traditional inpatient training, he interviewed for a
family practice residency. Family medicine was in its infancy at
the time and some believed the practice would soon die, but he
found what he was looking for in a family medicine residency at
McNeal in Berwyn, Illinois. He recalls, "I interviewed with Ken,
the residency director, who had a vision for family medicine that
inspired me. The decision to join him shaped my life's work."

In particular, two experiences at McNeal profoundly impacted
Martin's career direction. "During my first rotation in intensive
care, I had a heart attack patient who reminded me of my old
roommate and the situation with his mother. His near-death experience petrified him with fear. He wanted to hear about faith
issues, so we explored them and prayed together. My second
rotation came on the alcohol treatment unit. My passion found a
home that month."

*"We are going home to our-
selves. Going home to ourselves means accepting the
contours of our lives."*

— Robert Raines
Going Home (1985)

Martin credits his residency training as shaping his future in physician
health advocacies. The program was
unusual in its breadth of experience,
and a large part of the residency
training involved physician wellness.
He reports, "We received a grant in
1977-1978 to study the lifestyle of
physicians, investigating the impact
it has on patient care. The staff went through preventive medicine health evaluations, were introduced to alternative medicine, and were all given Shiatsu massages."

"I also spent 2 weeks at the Family Institute in Chicago studying
Family Systems Theory. Later at an international conference,
Rachel Naomi Remen, MD, spoke about how medical training
damages physicians. After hearing her, I wrote Ken, thanking him
because my residency was just the opposite, an inspiring 3 years.
In the early 1970s, he pioneered all that has become so important in
medicine today: preventive medicine, holistic care, alcoholism,
behavioral health, alternative medicine, and geriatrics. Even
structured into the residency program were 2 months working in
a Scottish home taking care of elderly patients."

Continuing, he says, "The seeds of what we know today as care management were planted back then. Ken had criteria cards for every office visit. The charts were audited, and all went into the computer in terms of three types of visits: acute care, care of chronic illness, and preventive medicine. If, as a resident, you didn't have at least 25% of your practice devoted to preventive medicine you were called on the carpet. Health appraisal was used as a tool to teach preventive medicine. Looking back, I am even more awestruck by this approach," he admits.

Martin's passion for working with recovering alcoholics serves as the current focus of his life in medicine. "I had an aunt who was an alcoholic," he shares. "When I was a first-year medical student, my uncle called asking me to come up to Indiana. She was in the hospital and didn't have a clear diagnosis. I hadn't even seen one patient, so how could I help, but I made the trip. A classic, upper-middle class closet alcoholic, I discovered she had the DTs after visiting with the staff. She was close to me, almost like a second mother, but got no treatment and, immediately after leaving the hospital, began drinking again. Desperately ill and becoming more and more isolated, nobody had any idea how to help her."

"When you have that kind of thing in your family," he explains, "you start looking for answers in your own studies. I took care of many alcoholics in medical school and I didn't see one single person recover. No one ever talked about how to help them and there were a lot of really negative attitudes toward such patients in general. So at the time, I saw no hope for my aunt."

As Martin completed his residency, his director observed his intense passion helping alcoholics recover and offered him a job on the faculty of the family residency program, as well as the medical directorship of the alcohol treatment center. Again, the experience helped shape his future.

He recalls, "When I got to the treatment center, I met my first recovering alcoholic, its director. For the first time, I witnessed people working as a team. The doctors didn't just bark out orders to be followed; they communicated with each other. And, it was the first place where people systematically addressed spiritual issues, a necessity because the center's philosophy of treatment was based on the 12 steps of AA. I found a team and an environment where I could apply my new knowledge about family systems. It crystallized my career."

"Fifty percent of my patients were recovering alcoholics and I became known as the doctor who knew what they valued the most, namely, the 12-step program. Even though not a recovering alcoholic myself, I practice the principles for my own spiritual growth. They did something for my own spiritual life that I hadn't found in my church. Since then, those two have come together for me."

Martin's aunt eventually accepted help, entering a treatment program and joining a support group. Although it meant a long drive from her home in Indiana to the center, she never missed a session and has been recovering for 25 years.

Like all physicians, Martin makes mistakes; a most cherished gift surfaced as a result of one. Referred to him by the administrator of the hospital where he worked in Chicago, a world-famous theologian from the University of Chicago became his patient. "I took care of him and his whole family," Martin says. "I cared for his wife through her breast cancer. After her surgery, I spoke with the cancer committee at the hospital about adjunctive therapies. I never was satisfied with the answers they gave, but failed to pursue my instincts. Later when the cancer metastasized I felt guilty that I hadn't gotten her to more treatment earlier. The theologian trusted me with his wife, whom he dearly loved. I felt I had failed him," he says emotionally. He recalls attending her memorial service and seeing the remembrance cards. "So, I wrote him a note, telling him about how disappointed I was that I (and medicine in general) couldn't have done more for his wife. I received a wonderful letter in return saying he didn't realize how much these kinds of disappointments affected physicians. It was very healing to receive his forgiveness personally and professionally."

"Today, I never hide mistakes. I can speak about them. Even though they are minor, I don't bury either the mistake or my feelings about it."

Martin eventually left McNeal and went to Parkside Medical at Lutheran General in Chicago. Notably a premier addiction treatment center, first locally and then nationally, Parkside attracted the best people. After about 2 years, he became medical director of the Parkside system.

"In that role, I evaluated health professionals and conducted many multidisciplinary assessments of high-risk people, including athletes and lawyers. I helped train a lawyer's assistance program on how to conduct interventions. I became involved with the Chicago police department and trained supervisors. Working with professionals became a sort of specialty. I also trained interveners for the state medical society's program." Eventually, the medical society requested that Martin direct their program. Currently, he serves as president-elect of the Federation of State Physician Health Programs.

"The wonderful thing," says Martin enthusiastically, "is I apply my passionate skills toward helping my colleagues, and through them, to reach other patients. It's been just wonderful to watch lives change."

He works primarily with recovering physicians, but he challenges the label calling them impaired. "I don't like to call them impaired physicians because the majority practice medicine with skill and safety in spite of their diagnosis. Their illnesses are in remission, and they are not in any way impaired," he explains. "Personally, I have epilepsy and heart disease, yet I practice everyday unimpaired. With the exception of a few, the same holds true for the physicians who are in our program. I am their advocate, convincing others that they are not impaired in spite of their diagnosis. They can be trusted to take care of patients just like any other physician. Many times, you hear stories about how they are better able to take care of patients because of their own recoveries."

He notes that with all the changes occurring in medicine today, the most common referrals are about physicians stressed out and coping poorly. "It gets labeled as 'disruptive behavior' or 'angry outbursts,' but, basically, these are people not coping very well with all the accelerating change in health care."

According to Martin, 80% to 90% of physicians' reactions spring from their childhood experiences. An April 2000 conference on physician stress, diagnosis, and management, highlighted the importance of one's personal history behind such reactions. He notes, "We see many physicians who are blind to damaging experiences until they enter therapy."

"Personally, I had a wonderful opportunity to gain such insights earlier in my career," Martin explains. "I realized that a lot of my reactions to the medical system, and especially toward the director of medical education at McNeal, resulted from my relationship to my father. I resolved that situation and am very grateful it happened before his heart attack at age 60.

He was healthy one day and dead the next. There was no saying good-bye."

"Many doctors react strongly to the changes in medicine, to authority figures, or to patients who cause them grief," he adds. "I came to understand such reactions through the family systems model. Today, we are starting a support group for such doctors and you don't have to have an addiction diagnosis to participate. I'm initiating it for myself as well as for others."

"For example," Martin relates, "I received a call from a physician greatly disturbed because the entire administration underwent change at the hospital where he practiced. This inner-city hospital faced continuing financial decay. He was called in and informed his contract was being canceled, his secretary was now working for the hospital, and to consider entering private practice."

At the time, Martin faced a related experience. "Two weeks before that contact, I had to convey a very similar message to our own medical group. I'm on the executive council and work half time as medical director at the Advocate Medical Group, a 270-member physician organization. Like most hospital-based groups, we've been losing money to the point where the system couldn't tolerate it anymore. So all contracts were terminated, and then they were reissued to most of the physicians, but not all. They downsized a little and cut compensation by anywhere from 10% to 30%, depending on the specialty. The corporate physicians from Advocate Health Care delivered the message on a Thursday morning. Then, as an executive council member, with considerable difficulty, I had to give my spin on it. We don't know exactly how many people are staying or going. During the transition, we are forming a group where we can talk and keep each other sane."

As with others whom we interviewed, we asked Martin to share his definition of the word *soul*. "For me," he explains, "soul is the spiritual part of me. It's that eternal part that will last beyond the end of my life. I am a soul in a body, not just a body with a soul." He also believes spirit and prayer powerfully serve the healing process. And, his faith offers guiding principles enabling him to stay resilient in times of change, both professionally and personally.

Unfortunately, largely because of managed care, Parkside deteriorated from being nationally and internationally known. He recounts, "In the language of the business of medical management, my passion became a 'dog.' But, I was able to cope by learning new knowledge and skills and receiving the gift of participating in the medical society's program."

Continuing, he says, "Even more profound was the setback to my personal health. I had been healthy all my life. The year I turned 40, along with my two college buddies, I participated in my first triathlon in Chicago. Even my e-mail address was TriathDoc," he grins. "I was fit and able to ignore my elevated cholesterol until, in 1997, I developed chest pain on one of my morning runs. I was angry with myself and disappointed with my family physician. I was robbed of my best stress management tool—running. I went to my church's fellow elders for prayer, then to a cardiologist for diagnosis and treatment recommendations. Then, we took a family vacation to process it all. I read, prayed, talked, processed, and came out with an 'aftercare agreement plan' for myself. When my cardiologist asked me why I was so relaxed during a catheterization, I knew it was because I had been the recipient of prayers by the elders."

Admittedly hopeful about the future of medicine, Martin says, "God's promises go beyond any circumstances. He has been faithful to me and to the vision for medicine I embody. Why give up hope now? Medicine is a gift. I want to be remembered as one who walked the path of recovery in my own life as an example of healing available to others."

Dancing Doctor

Rhonda Ringer, MD, MPH

For Dr Rhonda Ringer, preventive medicine consultant, passion for the profession of medicine means waking in the morning excited about helping someone and motivating that person to achieve healthy living. It represents a very satisfying joy emerging from within a person. Rhonda says it involves saying, "Ah, this is why I went into medicine. I would rather be doing this than anything else." She enjoys seeing people gain insight into themselves, creating passion and excitement in their lives. "When a patient comes to my office, I attempt to find something about them beyond a physical problem or complaint," she relates warmly. "It's that something touching the soul."

"One lady brought her aging mother to me because she was developing Alzheimer's disease. Her mother simply wanted to remain in bed all of the time and refused to take her medicine. During the process of taking her history and physical, I found out that her mother used to love to dance. At the end of the evaluation, she stood up rather painstakingly. I grabbed her hands and said, 'Louise, let's dance.' You should have seen her smile and the sparkle in her eyes. She grabbed my hands and we danced around the room. Her daughter then commented that she had not seen her mother so happy in years. Then we went into the hallway and did a little dance together for the office staff," she laughs.

"Several visits later, the mother commented, 'Doctor Ringer, we have to dance again.' I had forgotten the first incident, but here was a lady with Alzheimer's reconnecting to her passion that forever changed the way she felt about visiting our office. So, I seek to find something about people that excites them, whether it is dancing, a pet, a person, or a hobby. It helps to take their minds off of the concern that brings them to a doctor in the first place. Whatever I do for people medically seems to be augmented by such excitements. I would not want to practice medicine without attempting to uncover such passions of the soul." And, she believes it is the combination of using the best of scientific knowledge with what a physician knows about a patient's story that creates healing and is the mark of a good physician.

Rhonda's physician father served as her role model. She was about 10 years old when he began medical school.

"I developed an incredible interest in the profession, actually quizzing my father for his exams," she recalls. "I found it to be fascinating; so, I believe I have an innate bent toward this career. Also, as a teenager, I remember watching a program on television portraying actual footage from a vascular surgery where they were opening up the carotid artery of a person who was destined for a stroke. I saw them extracting some plaque and I said to myself, 'Wow! That's what I want to do.' It became a very strong motivator for me. I saw that you could take someone destined for trouble or death and, with one procedure, restore them to health again."

In addition to her clinical skills, Rhonda believes she brings many other talents to her practice. She loves to bring people together and especially make them laugh. Specifically, she is interested in studies showing the positive effect of laughter upon healing, documenting neurochemical changes that occur. A hands-on physician, she touches her patients as much as possible, and not simply as a part of conducting a physical. "I believe that touching bonds people to one another," she exclaims.

"I'm also a very spiritual person. In all of the histories that I take, I include a spiritual inventory. From the beginning, I understand their orientation, so it may become an arena where we can connect. It seems to be very meaningful to people. It helps them to understand that their doctor also has this orientation. I pray with my patients when appropriate and when I feel led to do it.

"We also have about four or five what I call spiritual prescriptions that I hand out along with medical prescriptions. Many of my patients find this quite meaningful, connecting mind, body, and spirit." Each spiritual prescription is a small card with a photograph from nature. One such example shows a waterfall on the front with the words "Especially For You." On the reverse side, it reads, "Prayer changes everything, and I want you to know that I have offered a personal prayer for you today." A verse from Isaiah 54:10, follows: "For the mountains may depart and the hills disappear, but My Kindness shall not leave you. My promise of peace for you will never be broken, says the Lord who has mercy upon you."

"When all is said and done, the essence of medical practice—'Medicine'—will always be a transaction of intimacy between two human beings."

— Ways, Engel & Finkelstein
Clinical Clerkships (2000)

Although Rhonda began practicing medicine in 1987, most of her career was in academic medicine. Less than a year before our interview, she opened her first clinical practice in the Women's Health Center at Celebration Health, Florida. The shift in focus from academic medicine to having a clinical practice came with mixed blessings.

"When I was in academic medicine teaching family health, there were two things I loved," she says smiling. "I loved to see the lights come on in young physicians' eyes when they 'got' something and I loved the challenge and excitement of a case." Enjoying the opportunity academic medicine afforded in the combination of research and medicine together, Rhonda delighted in being presented with a challenging and a diverse set of medical problems. The switch from academics to clinical practice was not without some pain, however. Sadly, she admits that practicing at Celebration Health, 45 miles from her home, required her to give up inpatient medicine and delivering babies. "This was hard." But, she adds, enthusiastically, "I have discovered the challenge in outpatient medicine."

However, some of her setbacks occurred around being financially successful in a managed care world. As a relatively new facility, the hospital carries tremendous overhead expense. She confesses to wrestling with the financial feasibility of her practice.

"I am currently considering whether it is financially feasible for me to continue my practice in family medicine," she states. "It's been very difficult because I've built close relationships with my patients, and I would hate to leave them. Also, everything I had ever dreamt about in a practice may not be practical in today's managed care environment. So far, I have survived by talking to a number of my colleagues who are feeling the same crunch. I also pray about it, looking for guidance and direction."

It is the paperwork and authorizations related to managed care that most bore her in her practice. "They steal valuable time that could be better utilized to assist people. I have spoken to many colleagues recently who are seriously considering career changes in some fashion because of these very issues," she reports sadly.

After much soul-searching and prayer, Rhonda appears to have found some degree of comfort in her decision making, releasing the struggle between the love of her practice and financial reality. Believing she has found an answer, she smiles, "To date, it strongly appears that I should continue in primary care, not looking to make a significant income but touching a large number of lives. The financial chips will have to fall where they may, and I will have to do the best I can to survive. But," she points out, "managed care and whole person medicine are not very compatible."

Reflecting on her comments, we felt an even stronger commitment to writing this book and getting it into the hands of the public. As have the many other physicians interviewed, Rhonda serves as an excellent example of a physician who is totally dedicated to her philosophy of health care and to her vocational calling. As mentioned in the introduction and elsewhere in this book, James Hillman claims, "Each person bears a uniqueness that asks to be lived and that is already present before it can be lived."[10]

Like most physicians, over the course of her medical career, Rhonda knows she has changed. "I am different today in the sense of realizing medicine as a calling and not just a job with a certain amount of prestige and income," she says. "As most physicians know, both of those latter factors are diminishing. Those who survive in this current climate see medicine as much more than a job. It demands so much time, energy, and emotion. We must process very intimate information, and we carry this knowledge in a very caring and gentle way, sometimes making life-and-death decisions."

In the midst of the demands of medicine and the changing health care environment, Rhonda finds hope in interacting with her patients. She sees them respond in a very positive and healing manner. In return, they find in her a special type of care. She is hopeful the public will eventually become a positive catalyst for changing the current system, standing up for their rights. Her personal outlook remains balanced between optimism and pessimism. "Unfortunately," she declares, "there is so much bureaucracy, business, and politics involved that I'm not sure the system will be allowed to right the wrongs."

Rhonda concludes our interview by expanding on developing her sense of trust that God will put her where she can be best utilized. "Sometimes I become anxious and want to throw up my arms in despair, especially about managed care. But, God put this passion for medicine inside of me, so I need to trust that I will be placed where I can best deliver my skills and not worry about future results," she maintains firmly. Subsequent to our interview,

---

[10] Hillman. *The Soul's Code.* New York, NY: Random House; 1996: 6.

Rhonda has embarked on a new journey, becoming a preventive medicine consultant.

Her words remind us of the Sufi saying to basically "show up, be present, and don't worry about the outcome." Such advice is easy to verbalize but quite difficult to follow. The Sufis also advise us to speak only after our words have managed to pass through three gates. At the first gate, we ask ourselves "Are these words true?" If so, we let them pass on; if not, back we go. At the second gate we ask, "Are the words necessary?" At the last gate, we ask, "Are they kind?"

The Joy of Home Care

Thomas Cornwell, MD

D r Thomas Cornwell experienced a twofold banner year in
1998. In some ways, two prestigious awards validated his
career path. In May, the American Academy of Home Care
Physicians bestowed the honor of House Call Doctor of the Year.
Then, in October, Tom was named by the Best Practice Network
as one of seven Heroes in Healthcare in the Chicago area. We
began our interview talking about his work. As he says,
"Literally, medicine is something I cannot not do."

Tom's road to becoming a physician was not a straight one.
His work can be viewed as the culmination of things falling
into his lap.

"I actually went to a Lutheran college thinking of becoming a
pastor," he relates. "There are no doctors in my family, but many
Lutheran ministers. But, I was just much more gifted at science
than I was at philosophy, theology, and especially public speaking," he says grinning. "When one of my advisors advised me
against the ministry, suggesting medicine as a better fit, I eventually agreed. Medicine became a natural place to combine my love
of science while at the same time helping people," he recalls.

As mentioned elsewhere, in *The Power of Myth*, Bill Moyers asks
Joseph Campbell, "Do you ever have the sense when you are following your bliss, as I have at moments, of being helped by hidden hands?" Campbell replies, "All the time."[11]

Throughout our conversation, Tom also expressed amazement
how hidden hands seem to have guided him. "Looking back at
my faith," he underscores, "I wonder how much God guided me
and what just happened."

"I did very well in medical school and ended up being selected
the outstanding graduate of my class. As is often the case in medical schools that are based in teaching care centers, I was dis-
suaded from going into family practice. It was as if I would be
throwing all my potential away. There were no family practice
electives open in the beginning of my fourth year. I applied to

---

[10] Campbell J. *The Power of Myth*. New York, NY: Doubleday; 1988: 120.

combined medicine-pediatric programs thinking this would make me a more 'academic' primary care doctor. One family practice program received permission to have one additional student and they 'happened' to call me to see if I was still interested. I loved the entire month and decided to go into family practice. Had the position not been created and had they not called me, I would not have gone into family practice, which I love."

"I will work in my own way, according to the light that is in me."

— Lydia Maria Child

At the conclusion of his residency, some personal problems led him to work in an emergency department for a year and then move on to Central DuPage Health's Immediate Care Centers. "With the stress of what was happening in my personal life, I didn't feel good about taking on the stress of starting a practice. Again, it was something unplanned."

In the early 1990s, Tom volunteered in an inner city clinic and then went on a short-term medical mission trip to Africa. Both experiences changed his focus. During this period, he continued working in an immediate care center, later serving as its director. He began to realize that, although the center offered financial stability, it provided little sense of mission.

"Intuitively, I felt drawn to the inner city where I could make more of a difference. My passion centers around helping the disenfranchised," he says emphatically. "In the inner city, people were disenfranchised from getting medical care because they didn't have insurance, only public aid. Today, my homebound patients have coverage but they are disenfranchised due to the inability to get to medical care. This is why we visit them at home."

Eventually, while continuing to work at the immediate care center, he was approached to join a new program called Call Doc, a physician house-call service. Because of his inner city volunteer work and mission experience, he was regarded as a perfect candidate to be its first physician. "Again," Tom says, "no intentionality was involved. It just fell into my lap."

When Joseph Jaworski published his book, *Synchronicity*, Tom read it with tears in his eyes because it reflected his own journey. Son of Watergate prosecutor Leon Jaworski, Joseph states, "We've all had those perfect moments, when things come together in an almost unbelievable way, when events that could never be predicted, let alone controlled, remarkably seem to guide us along our path." [12]

Tom continues, "We started the program, but after about 2 years, we began having significant financial problems, and this is where synchronicity arises. In the fall of 1995 and before the financial difficulties arose, I had asked a very successful business-man and his wife from our church to mentor my second wife and me. He could not meet with us until that January, and by then, the financial problems emerged making the program's continua-tion uncertain. We couldn't afford our rent and were behind thou-sands of dollars."

"Knowing that we were making such a difference in people's lives but uncertain about the viability of our future, when we finally met, I began to cry, relating our dilemma. Coincidentally, the man owned an unoccupied building that was for sale and he let the practice move in."

"Now, how many people do you know who invite you for din-ner just happen to own a building?" Tom asks. "Because it had been a Shell Oil Company facility, it had two huge garages for vehicles, so there was sufficient space. It was just amazing."

Still, the path was not smooth. "We moved, but continued to have financial problems. My wife and I used some of our per-sonal savings to help keep the practice going. We relied on her income for our own expenses since I was not getting paid. But, with our first child on the way and my wife resigning her posi-tion to stay home with the baby, the situation needed to change. I thought of quitting during those difficult days. Instead, I went back to my former employer, Central DuPage Health, and asked if they would be willing to support a house-call program. They enthusiastically agreed, which was the best thing that could have happened. The difficulties turned into a blessing."

Ultimately, the new organization, HomeCare Physicians (HCP) became a division of CENTRA, Central DuPage Health's group medical practice, supported by the system and Central DuPage Hospital Auxiliary. Tom currently serves as HCP's med-ical director.

To date, Tom's practice has made 10,000 house calls to more than 1,900 homebound patients. HCP's work received local media coverage with articles appearing in all Chicago area newspapers.

---

[12] Jaworski J. *Synchronicity: The Inner Path of Leadership*. San Francisco, CA: Berrett-Koehler; 1996: ix.

National publications highlighting HCP included *HomeCare Magazine*, *American Medical News*, *Medical Economics*, and *Physician Financial News*. A nationally televised PBS show featured Tom in May 1999, and WGN and CLTV highlighted him in early 2000. He was also on the local NBC affiliate.

"Physical presence always has a spiritual component; a patient's experience with sickness and death is somehow both shameful and endearing, degrading and ennobling. It moves one to prayer, if one is so moved."

— David Schiedermayer, MD, FACP

Pocket Guide to Managed Care (1996)

Tom beams when he talks about involvement with patients. His faith serves as the foundation for patient relationships. He recalls the first time he prayed with a patient, admitting that he prayed because he didn't know what else to do.

"It began," he reports, "in the inner city clinic where I was working. I had never talked to patients about prayer or read anything about if and when it was appropriate. But then, a stressed-out grandmother caring for her grandchildren came to me. The children's mother could not help out because, as a bystander, she had been shot during a gang fight. I was shocked, and not knowing what else to do, I suggested that we pray together."

"Later, a 17-year-old woman appeared at the clinic with zero emotion and eyes like rocks, almost catatonic. She had been horribly gang raped. I remember praying with her, saying, 'God, how can you let this happen?' I recall opening my eyes at the end of the prayer and seeing a tear sliding down her face and light reflecting off her eyes. She began coming back on a weekly basis and I saw how these visits were having a dramatic, positive impact on her. It doesn't take very many such experiences to realize the presence of a power existing beyond ourselves, accessed through prayer."

Because it had a Christian orientation, the health center became a relatively safe place to include prayer. He recalls many tears of appreciation from patients.

Since those first experiences of praying with patients, Tom routinely asks patients about their faith orientation during initial consultations. Today, he uses the extensive research now available documenting the impact of prayer upon healing when addressing conferences on the subject. "Surprisingly," he states, "physicians are less interested in the evidenced-based medical studies I offer than in the stories and pictures of the people who have been impacted by prayer."

On the subject of soul, Tom spoke specifically about how soul embraces a value system and the reality that much of our culture values money as an end in and of itself.

"What is going to make you happy? It's nice to have possessions and money, but in my opinion, ultimately, they don't foster much joy in life." Sadly, he notes, some physicians don't know the joy they are robbing themselves and their patients of by making it [medicine] often times more a business than a profession. Everyone's losing. And, I think the doctors are losing more than the patients."

As mentioned elsewhere, along with other qualities, soul values connectedness and intimacy. If money is used to these ends, then it will enhance our experiences of soul. In the book *Money, Money, Money*, Lynne Twist comments, "I see money a little bit like water. When water is moving and flowing, it cleanses, purifies, creates growth, and makes things green and beautiful. When it starts to slow down and is held still, it becomes stagnant and toxic."[13]

Returning to our conversation on patient care, Tom says he finds his work immensely satisfying and filled with amazing stories of wonderment. He recalls one woman he visited early in his work who was dying. Nothing else could be done for her. One day, he simply sat down, held her hand, and softly told her it was okay to leave this earth. She died while in the grip of his hand. Enormously grateful, the woman's daughter phoned saying they asked people to give money to his group rather than giving flowers. It was especially appreciated because it was during the time of greatest financial struggle.

On another occasion, a 20-year-old woman came to the immediate care center suffering with what Tom assumed were problems related to stress. "She had dozens of complaints sounding

---

[13] New Dimensions Foundation. *Money, Money, Money.* Carlsbad, CA: Hay House; 1998: 44–45.

stress-related," he remembers. "She had been to two neurologists and three psychiatrists, all of whom diagnosed her as having stress-related problems. She came to me about 7:00 in the evening and I thought to myself, 'After five specialists, what does she think this doctor is going to do?' I discussed with her that the definition of stress is any change—good or bad. I asked her if there were any changes happening in her life. It turned out she was leaving the next day to be a missionary in Europe. She had not mentioned this to any of the other doctors because she could not conceive of it as being stressful. Her parents had been missionaries in Europe, and she knew God would take care of her. She was not conscious of the stress, but the stress was manifesting itself through physical problems. Miraculously, no one else came into the center for one hour, allowing us to talk and pray. Reassuring her, I said, 'God sent you here tonight, and we'll take care of you.'" Looking back, Tom is convinced that of all the places she could have gone that night, there was a reason she came to the center.

"I have also witnessed miracles," Tom says excitedly. One story particularly came to mind. "A lady living in a nursing home had an ultrasound revealing a renal mass that was surely cancer. She decided she did not want to engage in invasive treatment, but to return to her apartment and wait for death. I was called to care for her. One day, I found her leg on the affected side swollen twice the size of her other leg. I suggested she should see an oncologist because the tumor might have invaded the lymph nodes. And, we prayed together."

Tom recalls praying, "God, either make her better or take her home to you, but don't make her suffer like this." Tom admits, "In my scientific mind, I hoped for death because a cure wasn't going to happen. However, when she eventually visited an oncologist, he discovered the swelling in her left leg was completely gone. A new CT scan showed the mass in her belly had also disappeared. This was a medical miracle."

"I don't really expect miracles," he confesses. "It's not common, but sometimes people heal even when faced with impossible odds. In any case, on a weekly basis at least, I continue to experience wonder, which is why I couldn't stop practicing medicine. It not only impacts our patients, but the lives of professional caregivers as well."

"In medical school," Tom relates, "we were taught to isolate emotion from the episode. I suppose to a degree it is necessary, because you go from one horrible situation in the ICU to another. We've been taught that it's dangerous to become emotionally involved; it will cause burnout. I probably do have more pain because of the increased intimacy with my patients. But, I also have much more joy," he adds emotionally. "I see patients pass away and I suffer, but there is also tremendous joy in terms of being part of their lives."

INNOVATORS

"Imagination is more important than knowledge."
—Albert Einstein

Assisting Living

William H. Thomas, MD

Picture a man, frail and bedridden, sleeping peacefully while a bird perches on his forehead. Envision an elderly woman, wrinkled by age, cuddling and rocking an infant while other children from a nearby child-care facility roam the halls, socializing with the residents of a nursing home. Imagine these same residents tending to vegetation throughout the building and cultivating a garden just outside its walls. This is an Eden Alternative™ facility in Bremerton, Washington, one of hundreds across America and beyond our borders dedicated to empowering and enlivening the elderly, and eliminating the plagues of loneliness, hopelessness, and boredom.

The concept for the Eden Alternative™ has its roots in a 1991 pilot project initiated by Dr Bill Thomas and seeded with a grant from the state of New York. According to Bill, it is more than just fuzzy props, potted plants, and the presence of children. It's about giving people a reason to live, an approach that also impacts the bottom line. In upstate New York, the original Eden Alternative™ pilot home saw a 26% reduction in turnover of nurses' aides, and a 50% drop in residents' infection rates. Meanwhile, the project's medication costs fell while those at a control facility rose during the same period. In a Texas facility, there was a 33% reduction in the use of PRN medications for anxiety and depression, a 44% decline in staff absenteeism, and a 60% cut in inhouse decubitus ulcers. In Milwaukee, a center reported their staff turnover rate 51% lower and the use of restraint dropped from 123 to 40 for an average population of 220 residents.[1]

Bill explains how his work as a physician evolved in this direction. "After beginning my work in a nursing home, it quickly became obvious that just prescribing drugs was not going to cut it for these people. I witnessed the slow, agonizing death of good people who suffered from an emptiness of spirit. They felt they had no reason to live. The problem wasn't about sufficient medical treatment, but about fulfillment in life. Nursing homes have long tended to confuse fulfillment with busyness. So, we began to experiment with alternative approaches, infusing the environment

---

[1] Reported at http://www.edenmidwest.com, September, 2000.

with huge numbers of plants, animals, and children. It included a radically redefined relationship between management and staff. The goal was to create an environment that was warm, suffused with life, laughter, and song in a natural, everyday manner, but not as an organized, structured activity. We came to call this approach the Eden Alternative™."

Today it is being practiced all over the world. More than 230 homes in North America implement the philosophy. Bill regards it as a social movement. He believes that the world can be made a better place by innovatively caring for frail elders. If this can be accomplished, it offers important lessons for society in general. In reality, the way we care for our elders mirrors the health of our culture. He reports, "One of the most important things elders have to teach us is about how to create a truly human society. A society caring for frail, elderly people in a tender and compassionate way is a better society in general. If we keep our promise to them, we actually make a better life for ourselves."

As mentioned during another interview, Rachel Naomi Remen, MD, informs us that dying people can teach us how to live well. Bill suggests that another way to frame this is to say that you can learn how to live by learning how to live in a healthy way with frailty in old age. Someone who can do this tends to be successful in a human and spiritual sense.

Bill originally began his college training by attending State University of New York at Cortland where he enrolled in a health education program. He remembers a spring day in May, sitting in a lecture listening to the professor speaking about measuring blood pressure. "I scribbled notes like crazy until she ended the lecture by saying that, of course, none of you will ever be doing this," Bill says. "I remember walking out of class that morning, saying to myself, 'Why can't I be a doctor?' It occurred to me for the first time that such a career was possible. So, I changed my major and completed the requirements for pre-med, graduating with a degree in biology."

It was quite interesting to jump from a state school to Harvard. Bill says surprisingly, "What helped me a lot in getting into the school was my involvement in politics. I was the president of the student association in college and also ran for the mayor of the city of Cortland. I didn't win the mayoral race, but had a good time making politics a part of my work." Bill graduated from medical school in 1986, followed by a residency in family medicine at the University of Rochester.

Subsequently, Bill began working in a little rural emergency department, a 30-bed hospital with a 3-bed ER and 2-bed ICU. "I really enjoyed the sense of being on my own," he reports. "I also did some work developing software for emergency rooms. In particular, I developed software that could analyze the waiting times for patients. It wound up being used all over the country."

In 1991, Bill began working in a nursing home. At first, he considered it to be a side job and not too serious. However, it soon became his greatest passion in life. He gave up the ER practice and committed all of his energy to long-term care. He served as medical director and at the same time was responsible for all of the patient care.

Passionate about medicine and his work, Bill states enthusiastically, "Today is the best time ever to be in the field of medicine. What we are living through today will be seen as the greatest challenge to the genuine soul of the profession of medicine. It bugs me when I hear doctors complaining like they have some kind of right to a golden age environment when all of America bowed to the 'wisdom' of the profession. Today, the excitement surrounding medical practice involves the reinvention of the profession. The decisions we make today will affect generations of doctors to come. Therefore, it is of vital importance to stand together for what is right and good, understanding that this kind of advocacy comes with honor and prestige of being a social, cultural institution. In our society, physicians are and will remain moral leaders in the community."

"When we exercise moral leadership, the whole profession looks and feels differently. When we act like aggrieved parties in a contract dispute, we diminish our profession and ourselves. We should help young physicians see the importance of moral leadership."

Bill believes having the best of all worlds means coming to terms with the holistic nature of good medical practice. He underlines, "One of the pillars of our profession, William Osler, is remembered as the consummate allopath, but he was really a holistic practitioner. Holistic thinking is ancient. Hippocrates would recognize holistic thought as being at the heart of the healing arts. Holism is too often confused with 'alternative' remedies.

In truth, it is a commitment to healing that is broad, deep, and inclusive. In fact, this is what the public wants from us. The medical profession falls from favor when it favors the technical dimension over the art of medicine. We can reclaim the mantle of healing and society is ready to give it to us, but we will have to earn it back."

Again, he informs us, "The real action is in the art of medicine. True, every year we will invent new drugs for a variety of conditions and I'm glad for this, but the vast uncharted plain ahead of us is not in pharmacological research but in how we conduct ourselves as physicians in the human community."

As Bill developed the Eden Alternative™ concept, he searched for a name that would reflect its nature. He took the name from the ancient story of Eden, suggesting, "If you study the myths of origin, you find that many cultures have stories of ancient times where humans live in gardens. Eden is the best known of these. The idea that humans were actually meant to live in a garden provides colorful imagery. In nursing homes, we wanted to create an alternative to the medical, scientific institution of today. To do this, we envisioned people living in a garden-like environment. Somewhat ironically, we don't need fancy technology or multimillion dollar grants to make this happen. It can come about in any facility in any community in the world. The answers are all around us."

To learn more about the Eden Alternative™ environment, we visited with Lori Colwell, the administrator of the nursing home in Bremerton, Washington, that embraces this approach. With many different kinds of birds, animals, and vegetation on site, the regulators had just finished an inspection of the facility and found zero defects. That's not easy, Lori commented, because nursing homes place second only to nuclear power plants in terms of the complexities of regulations.

We [the authors] experience the Eden Alternative™ movement as one creating sacred, soulful space for people. Consequently, we asked Bill to share his perspective about the meaning of soul.

"It is that which makes us human," he claims. "Physically, we are nitrogen, phosphorus, carbon, and other elements. We possess DNA, neurons, and synapses, and so on, all of which are very common in the national work. However, for me, soul represents that untouchable, unknowable mystery that makes us human. Soul is irreducible."

Of course, we take the nature of soul a step further, believing that it manifests itself, not only in humans, but also in the entire environment. In his book, *Care of the Soul*, Thomas Moore speaks of soul as engaging the vernacular, manifesting itself in things and in places that increase our sense of the sacred.[2] For this reason, we view an Eden Alternative™ facility as especially enhancing soul. If you were to walk into such a place, you would sense that it has a personality of its own. Or to state it in negative terms, while clean, such a building and its atmosphere are not antiseptic. It is not bland, without color, pictures, plants, or even animals.

> "[Sacred] space speaks of caring, of quiet, of compassion. Grief, exhaustion, fear, and even confusion are there as well. There is candor and inquiry, but overarching all are love and respect for human life."
>
> — Clif Cleaveland, MD
> *Sacred Space* (1998)

Bill also concurs with Thomas Moore that soul requires deep intimacy. He declares, "One of the things we talk about is fostering intimacy between staff and residents. This goes against the grain of keeping professional distance. Of course, there are certain potential problems with this approach. Intimate relationships between people can get complicated. But it's that which is worth living for. So, staff listens to the stories of the elders and, in turn, we share our stories with them."

"Here is a distinction we make in terms of providing health care. When treatment is provided for an individual [for something] such as a broken leg, a screw can be placed in the leg without ever knowing the person's name, and certainly not his/her story. However, if we are going to take care of a person, we must know that individual's story."

In Mitch Albom's beautiful book titled *Tuesdays with Morrie*,[3] the author spends Tuesdays with his beloved college professor as he is dying from cancer. Mitch speaks about his deep love for Morrie as he tells the story of his life and his profound wisdom and insight. This is what establishing an intimate relationship with elderly residents and listening to their stories means. And, you don't have to be a college professor; every person's story is unique and extraordinary.

[2] Moore T. *Care of the Soul*. New York, NY: HarperCollins; 1992.
[3] Albom M. *Tuesdays With Morrie*. New York, NY: Doubleday; 1997.

Bill continues, "On the other hand, in medicine, we often believe that if we have the facts, we can take care of people. That's not true. We must know their story as well."

As noted earlier in this book, we believe it is also important for the patient to know the physician's story. Agreeing with us, Bill responds with an animated "Yes!" giving the following example. "My wife Jude and I have five kids. Two of our girls have Otohala's Syndrome, a very devastating defect in brain development causing blindness and profound developmental delay. The fact that these girls are an important part of my life changes who I am as a person, how I practice medicine, and how I approach people with disabilities or who happen to be frail and elderly. If you wish to know who I am as a physician, you must know about my girls. It's not a footnote to our relationship. However, at least in the past, many physicians believed that such knowledge was irrelevant to the service they provided. In the future, such information will be quite relevant, whatever the nature of your story. Every human story is filled with victory, despair, joy, and loss."

As many physicians have shared with us, Bill also shares an experience of having a setback during his practice and how he dealt with it. With considerable emotion, he reports, "Wow, one of the most powerful events of my professional life occurred when I was working in the emergency room. An 18-year-old woman came to see me complaining about a cough. I examined her but could not find anything wrong. I gave her some advice for dealing with an upper-respiratory illness, asked her to follow up with her regular physician, and sent her home. About 1 week later, she reappeared in the ER in full arrest and I had to run a code on her. She died because she took oral contraceptives and developed a deep vein thrombosis, causing her to throw clots to the lung, resulting in respiratory problems. This was a shattering experience for me," he confesses. "I almost could not continue, feeling like I had fallen from a terrible cliff, that I had failed this woman in such a profound manner. Going back to work became the hardest thing I've ever done."

We asked Bill how he dealt with such pain and grieved this loss. "I sat in a dark room in a rocking chair for a long time," he says. "I'm sorry to say that I did not talk to any other physicians about my grief, nor did I share it with my family." We suggested to Bill that many physicians think they must be perfect. But from conducting other interviews, we feel that one characteristic of a good physician is the recognition that mistakes are part of the profession. "Yes," Bill replied, "that's the lesson that is seared on your soul and not something that can be transmitted in a med school lecture."

On the other side of the equation, Bill reports experiencing much mystery and wonder in his work. "I remember one time when I was in my family medicine residency," he states, "when I took care of pregnant women. I also worked in the pediatric ICU, one of those situations where you are up all night long and working for 24 hours. At 5 in the morning they brought in a 9-month-old child who had stopped breathing. We coded the infant, but she did not survive. We had to go out to the waiting room and inform the mother and father. Then, at about 9 am, I was released from duty and raced over to the office because, just a few days previously, I delivered a baby to a young mother who was giving the child up for adoption. I had to take the mother and the baby to a church where they would be seated in one room while the adoptive parents remained in another. My job was to carry the child from the birth mother to the adoptive parents. The birth mother and I discussed whether she was certain about her decision. When she assured me she was ready, I took the child from the arms of the birth mother, walked down the hall into the room of the adoptive parents, and placed the baby into the arms of the new mother."

"Afterward, I returned to the office to see patients and eventually went home at 6 pm. That evening, I remember thinking to myself, no other vocation could possibly give you the experiences of that day. So, in medicine, wonder continually permeates the atmosphere."

Two of Bill's heroes, both in the field of medicine, made a profound impact on him. "One of my heroes is Dr Jack Ringler, who was a senior resident when I was at Harvard. He appears to me as the greatest resident officer *ever*. He took the medical rotation and made it a joy. I'd follow that man anywhere. Another great hero of mine is T. Franklin Williams, a pioneer in the field of geriatrics who is the editor of the *Oxford Textbook of Geriatric Medicine*. He served as a role model for me and was someone I could turn to for advice in medicine and life in general."

As we ended the interview, Bill recounts his 1999 bus trip throughout America. He and his family took a month traveling 10,000 miles and visiting 27 cities teaching people about the Eden

Alternative™. He also performed a one-man, theatrical production based on a novel he wrote, called *Learning From Hannah*.[4] Inspired by events in Bill's own life, this fictional work presents his personal philosophy toward medicine and healing. The book tells of a place where the wisdom of the elders has built a life worth living for all. It remains to be seen how the world comes to accept such wisdom.

The following 10 principles stand at the heart of the Eden Alternative™:

1. The three plagues of loneliness, helplessness, and boredom account for the bulk of suffering in a human community.
2. Life in a truly human community revolves around close and continuing contact with children, plants, and animals. These ancient relationships provide young and old alike with a pathway to a life worth living.
3. Loving companionship is the antidote to loneliness. In a human community, we must provide easy access to human and animal companionship.
4. To give care to another makes us stronger. To receive care gracefully is a pleasure and an art. A healthy human community promotes both of these virtues in its daily life, seeking always to balance one with the other.
5. Trust in each other allows us the pleasure of answering the needs of the moment. When we fill our lives with variety and spontaneity, we honor the world and our place in it.
6. Meaning is the food and water that nourishes the human spirit. It strengthens us. The counterfeits of meaning tempt us with hollow promises. In the end, they always leave us empty and alone.
7. Medical treatment should be the servant of genuine human caring, never its master.
8. In a human community, the wisdom of the elders grows in direct proportion to the honor and respect accorded to them.
9. Human growth must never be separated from human life.
10. Wise leadership is the lifeblood of any struggle against the three plagues. For it, there can be no substitute.

---

[4] Thomas WH. *Learning From Hannah*. Acton, MA: VanderWyk & Burnham; 1999.

Pioneer Surgeon

Milton Weinberg, MD

Becoming a thoracic surgeon during the mid-1950s, Dr Milton Weinberg's early career was filled with wonder and excitement. Because thoracic surgery was in its relative infancy, he pioneered many of its procedures. As he says grinning, "My board number was in the 600s, whereas today there are more than 6,000 physicians in the specialty." He recalls that thoracic surgeons all knew each other quite well and national meetings were extremely exciting.

"As you can imagine," he says, "an awesome event occurred for me when for the first time, a patient's heartbeat was stopped in order to perform surgery; then afterward I got to see it resume pumping again. I never got over the wonder of this procedure; it was as exciting as anything I've experienced. There was always some apprehension involved. Of course, we surgeons are not supposed to have a lot of doubts, but there was always some concern," he admits.

"I remember a picture in *Life Magazine* depicting a heart transplant, a procedure that I have never performed. In the picture, there was a man holding up a jar containing his own heart. That's about as awe inspiring as it gets."

Milton's long career is filled with touching and sometimes humorous patient stories. "There was one lady who I will never forget," he recalls. "A fair number of patients report being awake during the surgery and later tell about hearing the surgery team speaking to one another. Others tell things that never really happened, as though they were dreaming. This woman was in trouble; her blood pressure was falling. We had to lighten the anesthesia in order to raise her pressure. We were talking to each other about what we were doing. Afterward, this woman quoted us word for word; she had been conscious, although fortunately she wasn't experiencing any pain."

"I also remember a little two-year-old boy who brought a Snoopy with him to the hospital. Everything we did to the boy, whether it was an IV or a chest tube, we first had to perform on the dog. Snoopy got the same dressings or whatever. I have photographs of both the boy and his Snoopy."

"Some occurrences were not really funny, but rather whimsical. I had a couch in my office where the family would sit, usually with a child. In this instance, midway into our conversation they began to smile, even though I was attempting to communicate some rather serious information. When I glanced at the child, I saw him mimicking my hand gestures. This happened to me a number of times during my years of practice."

Although in his 70s and retired from surgical practice, Milton remains active in the medical field. His changing career direction is a perfect example of the ability of talented physicians to transition into related positions, continuing to use their vast professional knowledge. His wonderful, ongoing relationship with a Chicago-area hospital grew into a unique position. In 1986 and nearing the age of 65, he was asked to engage in a specific project for the Lutheran General Hospital. Originally he assumed it would be a 2- or 3-year involvement, but the relationship has continued for more than 14 years.

"I had a trainee working for me and after a few years I thought he would take over running the program. Then the former chairman of the surgery department decided to step down. I became interim chairman and later, chairman. Then, various other tasks came my way. A few years ago I suggested that they find a replacement for me. They found one, but again, the new chairman requested that I stay on to help him. It's wonderful! It keeps me in the profession I love," he says enthusiastically. "It's very exciting, so I feel that I am about as lucky as I could be."

Milton continues, "I'm responsible for doing anything that makes the chairman's life easier. Today, there are many different kinds of auxiliary tasks needing to be accomplished. These include writing letters of recommendation, credentialing, and attending meetings for the head of the department. I also have committee responsibilities and review board accountabilities, so I am exposed to a considerable amount of research. The department of surgery has 11 divisions, including all of the surgical specialties except OB/GYN. I work in a robust environment. At my age, it's a great treat to be able to continue in the profession."

Milton loves medicine because it contains so much variety. It provides intellectual stimulation and he believes that if it is performed well, it can be all-consuming.

"I've had the privilege of being involved in many national activities," he tells us. "I was a representative to the AMA in thoracic surgery and to the AATS and on other national committees.

All of these activities added to the excitement. In addition, I was in practice for more than 35 years, not counting residency. When young people talk to me about the possibility of entering medicine, vocationally, I tell them there is nothing out there that can touch the profession. I performed pediatric cardiac surgery and interfaced with many families. It was wonderful to be trusted with the care of their children."

The young physicians he sees energize Milton. "Today, the young physicians entering the profession are wonderful. They are smart, capable, and you can see yourself reflected in many of them. I have an opportunity to associate with them through the medical education programs."

Milton was drawn into medicine because his father was a physician, and he never even considered a different career. He came from a small town in South Carolina, so the horizons of opportunity were not very broad. His father was one of two of the first urologists in the entire state.

Milton finished high school at the age of 16. As he tells us, with only 11 grades, he was in college and medical school before he knew what was happening to him. He gravitated to surgery because he was in training when new technology expanded the capabilities of cardiac surgery.

"When I was in clinical training," he says, "the first blue baby operation was performed. I saw a 3- or 4-year-old child who was deathly ill, unable to sit up or walk. After surgery, suddenly the child began to perk up and walk before leaving the hospital."

"We see soul as personal and unique—grounded in the depths of personal experience."

— Lee Bolman & Terrence Deal
Leading With Soul (1995)

Addressing the meaning of the word *soul*, Milton believes, "Soul is whatever it is that makes you a person. Every person I've ever met is unique." His perception parallels that of the Swiss psychologist C.G. Jung. His book, *Modern Man in Search of a Soul*, concerns the lifelong journey toward individuation, or toward simply "being oneself" apart from the collective norms of society. [5] Therefore, Milton describes at least one essential dimension of soul when he speaks of our uniqueness.

[5] Jung CG. *Modern Man in Search of a Soul*. New York, NY: Harcourt, Brace & World; 1933.

Like most physicians, Milton acknowledges changing over a lifetime of practicing medicine. "I certainly hope I have changed," he states emphatically. "A doctor doesn't mature much differently than other people. Along with acquiring a large amount of factual knowledge, we improve our ability to handle relationships, or at least I hope we do."

"On the other hand, the process of maturing includes not only the expansion of knowledge, but also the deterioration of certain skills. One of the reasons I stopped doing surgery was because of a loss of some of my physical skills. There came a point where my experience could no longer compensate for the loss of manual dexterity. Besides, I thought that some of the younger MDs were performing surgeries better than I, so I ended this part of my career. Some of the senior surgeons whom I greatly admired kept practicing surgery long after they should have stopped. I couldn't imagine putting myself in that position. I loved my practice, but there came a time to end it and go forward with my life in other ways. That happened at age 65. For a while thereafter, I assisted some of the younger surgeons, especially in the pediatric areas, but after a few years even this came to an end."

As we have with some of the other physicians interviewed, we asked Milton what he would like his patients to say about him professionally at the end of his life. After some reflection, he begins.

"First, of course, that I was a professional. After a diagnosis, I sometimes had to tell parents that there was a 10% or greater chance that their child would die during or after surgery. Occasionally they went for a second opinion, but more often they would say, 'Fine, doctor, we trust you.' For me, that is awesome. I hope I defined myself by recognizing the responsibility that came with that kind of trust. I felt that I had an obligation to behave in such a manner that generated and honored this trust. Even when things didn't go as hoped, I would want people to say that I fulfilled my obligations, that I did the best I could with the surgery and that I provided them with the best medical care available."

It has been said that different physician specialties exhibit particular characteristics. Some people claim that they can spot a surgeon when he or she walks into a room because of their demeanor. We've heard this described with various words such as "ego" or "self-confidence." Yet, most would say that if one has to have surgery, you want a physician who is supremely confident and without any doubts.

We asked Milton to respond to such observations. Agreeing with the observation, he said, "I have no problem with that perception. Particularly with thoracic and cardiac surgeons, I think that people in such specialties tend to be relatively self-assured. I know some people who have no doubts about anything, but I think that most of us, while being self-confident about our capabilities, have some doubts, especially with developments over which we have little or no control. We don't control everything and there are always variations in terms of what unfolds in an operation. It's the recognition that, while we attempt to be highly competent in our specialties, there are always uncertainties." Amplifying on that thought, he continues, "For example, during the very early days of introducing the heart/lung machine, the statistics indicated a 35 to 40% chance of having some brain damage."

Many physicians believe that healing is partly a physical process and partly mental. Affirming this belief, he states, "No one in surgery or in other medical specialties can grasp the mental and motivational dynamics of the healing process. Motivation is overwhelmingly important. My wife had her knee replaced and was given a walker to assist her mobility. She couldn't stand using it and discarded it almost overnight. She was so well motivated that she immediately began walking without such assistance. On the other hand, some patients may never fully recover because there are other issues involved in their makeup."

Milton shared a practice strategy he used to speed the recovery process. "I attempted to have new patients visit me in the office as soon as possible after leaving the hospital. Of course, right after surgery I informed them of the recovery process and what they could do to hasten it. But my patients were still stressed and perhaps frightened immediately after surgery, so I had them return to me so that I could reinforce what they could do to speed up the healing process."

Beyond this, Milton believes that prayer and spirituality play a part in healing. "My wife and I have a very close relationship with an Anglican minister. My wife is a member of his board. John asked me if I ever witnessed a miracle. Believing in them and witnessing them are two different matters. My response to him was negative. I've seen people with far-advanced cancer get well again. During my residency, I operated on a woman who had incurable cancer. After the surgery, we predicted that she would die in the near future. However, some 6 or 8 years later with no additional treatment, she was still living a full life. Her cancer had simply stopped growing. I would label this a mystery, but not necessarily a miracle."

"On the other hand," he continues, "you asked me about prayer. I think the best prayer is related to fulfilling God's purpose rather than praying for a specific cure, because that may not be what God has in mind for us. I don't know that much about them, but apparently studies are available showing the positive effects of prayer. I don't have the foggiest idea whether this is a consequence of the prayer or is caused by a person's will to live."

> "It is not in an arbitrary 'degree of God,' but in the nature of man, that a veil shuts down on the facts of tomorrow."
>
> —Ralph Waldo Emerson

During one of her courses at Southern Methodist University, Dr Ruth Barnhouse, whom we have mentioned a few other times in this book, addressed the issue of prayer and miracles. Two students in the class reported having relatives who were seriously ill. The class prayed for both of them. One relative quickly recovered from his illness and the other subsequently died. Thereafter, the obvious question emerged whether one set of prayers was answered and the other petitions denied. Ruth's perspective was similar to Milton's. Prayer, she maintained, is not pulling some divine string in order to get God's attention. We have at best a foggy perspective of how prayers are answered, let alone what happens to us after death. In the totality of God's purpose, we might assume that both prayers were answered, but not necessarily in accordance with our desire for continued life on earth.

Dr Barnhouse continued by describing a miracle as something mysterious that happens when time seems to speed up or slow down. For example, when someone rapidly recovers from an illness beyond all expectations and explanations, one might describe it as the miracle of time accelerating. On the other hand, when a supposedly terminally ill person lives far beyond all prospects, one might say that time slowed down considerably, particularly in terms of the spread of the disease.

Much is being said today about the stress involved in the current practice of medicine and its many responsibilities. We asked Milton how he thinks physicians handle such stress.

In terms of his own specialty, he says that he never looked upon it as being particularly stressful. It's both a job and a responsibility. Milton tells the story of an anesthesiologist friend of his who was hospitalized for a cardiac catheterization for investigation of angina.

"The night before, someone went into cardiac arrest right down the hall from him. He ran down the hall, grabbed the cart, and resuscitated the person with no problem, because that was his job and what he does every day. However, he was having difficulties in his family life. When he went home each night, the conflicts completely overwhelmed him, resulting in angina. Considering what they do every day, I don't see physicians as being stressed out. It's the rest of the stuff we have to deal with, such as HMOs, interpersonal conflicts, and especially, an atrocious legal climate for doctors."

Given his long, active medical career and his current unique position, Milton is enthusiastically optimistic about medicine's future. "Absolutely optimistic! In the 90s, I sat on the admissions committee at the University of Chicago, and the young people we had an opportunity to review were simply wonderful. They were bright, energetic, and just as idealistic as we were when we entered medical school. Of course, they are in a different social environment today than we were in my generation. But, again, I don't think there is any greater privilege than sitting in a room with a patient and being in a position to serve him or her. The mess that we face administratively today hopefully will be resolved. I would encourage people to enter the profession in a minute."

To the physicians who are in the middle of their careers today and who are feeling tired and frustrated, Milton says, "I would advise them to get a good office and office manager, then take care of anyone who walks through the door. When I was practicing with a partner, we told our office manager not to inform us whether a patient had insurance, was paying the bills, or was a no pay. That was not part of our business. We knew that we were doing all right financially and had a comfortable living. So, my advice to the younger doctors is simply to take care of anyone who walks through the door. Eventually, the financial rewards will come. The other rewards, which are infinitely more important and joyful, also will be present. In addition, the scientific developments emerging in medicine today will continue to make it a very exciting profession. The vistas are wide open."

Practicing Out of the Box

Lon M. Hatfield, MD, PhD

Our conversation with Dr Lon Hatfield began with his statement that earlier in his career he would never have imagined its current turn in direction. In family practice some 24 years, Lon opened his Healing Arts Center in northeastern Washington in 1998. With a twinkle in his eye, Lon confesses that he is a "recovering physician." Explaining, he continues, "For me, a lot of allopathic medicine just doesn't work and letting go of that 2 years ago to start a new program was a huge undertaking. I don't know why I was foolish enough to do that," he confides. "There's a lot of work involved."

Lon views himself not so much as a "doer" in the usual sense of the word, but as someone being led in this current direction. Some of the wisdom literature writers suggest, as does Ramesh Balsekar in his book, *A Net of Jewels: Daily Meditations for Seekers of Truth*, that our calling emerges when our passion intersects with some kind of void in the world.[6] We simply have to be present to it. As Lon says, "In this context, the center was just what was needed to fill a void."

Lon's deep passion for his work is evident in his reflections. Although he says that he doesn't have a clear definition of what passion means, he knows he is fully engaged and likes each moment of his work. He credits some force in the past as leading him in his current direction. Describing this feeling, he explains, "I love being present with each person in each moment, whether it is happy or tragic. I think I understand a little more now what Rupert Sheldrake means when he speaks of morphogenic fields, where something's pulling you into it as opposed to something pushing you into it." Lon identifies the feeling as "something coming to my attention, coming into a conscious awareness as though there is a purpose behind it." We liken it to what happens in the Northwest during summer weekends when people pile into the cars and head for the mountains, as though nature pulls them back to their roots.

For Lon, practicing medicine reflects this kind of pull, something he "cannot not do." His journey toward medicine began

---

[6] Balsekar RS. *A Net of Jewels: Daily Meditations for Seekers of Truth.* Redondo Beach, CA: Avaida Press; 1999.

when he was 12 years old. He remembers, "When I was 12 years old, I wrote a paper on what I would be when I grew up and it involved the general practice of medicine." Although unable to recall specific events, he suspects childhood experiences with his family physician probably played a part in his decision making. Lon recalls fond memories of that physician.

"I grew up in Des Moines, Iowa. My folks were divorced when I was 2 years old and my mother, who also taught school, raised me as an only child. Paul Gibson was my doc. Very personal, he was an incredibly wonderful individual who trained as an ear, nose, and throat physician. I still remember him assembling the hypodermic needle, filling it up with penicillin or whatever I had to have. Later, we'd go into his office adjacent to the exam room. He'd chat for a while with us and he would smoke a cigarette; at that time that was what docs did. My mother and I would just sit there and talk. We just loved this guy."

"As my mother grew older and her health deteriorated, Paul thought that wine would help her diet and increase her appetite. Of course, as a Methodist, she would have none of that." Lon laughs heartily as he recalls Paul's solution. "So, he would go to the store with his wife, Betty, buy Mogan David wine, and bring it to our house in a brown paper bag marked 'Medicine.' He was just marvelous."

Lon continues, "When I was in college, my mentor was the head of the chemistry department. He claimed that chemistry was much more intellectually stimulating than medicine and that I should switch majors. Honoring him and his vision, I went to graduate school at Purdue and received a PhD in biochemistry. However, I decided that I still had to pursue medicine."

Subsequently, he taught biochemistry in medical school and ran a research laboratory in the school's department of psychiatry. Lon decided that research was not his love. "I needed more connection with people. I then entered a residency program at Cedar Rapids, Iowa, allowing me to experience a broad base of medicine, including surgery and obstetrics."

Realizing that they could essentially settle anywhere they wanted after completing his residency program, Lon and his wife decided to investigate the Northwest where they had always enjoyed vacationing. They searched for a place where they could have some autonomy, and yet not so small that they wouldn't have a good education system for their kids. Eventually, they found Colville, Washington, a community they love and where they raised two daughters.

Lon finds his practice filled with wonder, but there have been setbacks as well. Lon laughs when he recalls opening their original multispecialty clinic. "Our office manager, who helped bring five different practices together, had a medical breakdown, and I had to put him in the hospital. Next, the driveway in the front of the clinic collapsed on the opening day. But," he says, "you just roll up your sleeves and do what has be done."

A number of years later, the clinic suffered some financial and management difficulties (as most clinics do at times), and Lon was installed as its president. Through his guidance, he was able to turn the financial picture around. Again referring to Ramesh Balsekar, Lon explains, "He says that what's going to happen is not in your hands. So forget about what is going to happen and do your duty."

Leaving an established clinical practice to open his Healing Arts Center required making a major decision and letting go of something he was convinced wasn't working the way he wanted it to. According to Lon, a progression of things ultimately led to his decision. "For about 18 years, I've helped people stop smoking through the use of acupuncture. I've counseled kids, provided homeopathic medicine, and given some supplements for several years. However, about 4 years ago, a naturopath doctor, who was one of my partners for a while, learned to do a procedure called Nambudripad's Allergy Elimination Technique (NAET). Developed by Devi Nambudripad in Los Angeles for people with allergies, it eliminates sensitivities in about 70% of people. Born in America, Nambudripad's parents migrated from India."

Lon confesses that he dismissed NAET initially. "I said, 'That's the goofiest thing I ever heard.' But, I sent a few people to him [Nambudripad] and they got better." Although he admits that he didn't understand the principles behind the treatment, he was impressed enough to travel to Los Angeles and learn NAET.

"I had 30 people who were guinea pigs. During the time we treated them, one didn't get better at all, 35% got better, and 65% got over their allergies completely. One patient was a psychotherapist who had a lot of food allergies. We treated her and the allergies vanished."

This is just one example of how Lon often operates outside the box of conventional medicine. His growing awareness that colleagues in his group were becoming uncomfortable with evolving interest in nontraditional medical methodologies, yet desiring to learn whatever was necessary to treat his patients effectively, led Lon to face a critical practice decision. He recalls realizing that he needed to learn more about this new direction he was exploring and he also felt the need to work on his spiritual life. He decided to embark on a 2-month sabbatical. It was during a study of neural therapy from Germany that he learned how the NAET system worked through the autoimmune system. And, during this period, he reached a turning point in his practice. "I realized that I couldn't live exclusively with the conventional model. It just didn't fit. Upon returning, my colleagues and I discussed offering alternative medicine within the clinic setting." In addition, for Lon, there was a deeper question. "Does my calling say that I've got to do something outside the clinic?"

Lon's increasing knowledge of nontraditional medicine led him to leave the clinic and open the Healing Arts Center. "My experience helped me to understand that Western medicine is far too restrictive to help people holistically who have significant major problems. Not excluding it [Western medicine], you have to get outside that box and begin using the things that help to really change a person's life."

Asked whether he is different today as a physician, he says, "When I started my practice, I could never have envisioned what I am doing today. However, I always have been a person who has had a curiosity about things. When something happens that I don't understand, it raises my curiosity. Also, having been in biochemistry research, I have a healthy disrespect for the establishment, realizing that it's very politicized. Of course, often unconventional practices become accepted over time."

Primarily, Lon's practice today is about out-of-the-box medicine. His patients' stories are testament to the results. One such nontraditional method the clinic offers is BodyTalk. Developed by Dr John Veltheim, it combines concepts from 5,000 years ago—TCM–Acupuncture, Chiropractic, Osteopathy, Neural Therapy, Kinesiology, and Reiki—to provide a faster way to do NAET and all the other body balancing procedures being used.

"I had a wonderful woman who was 69 years old who had a stroke. She was doing fairly well, but had no feeling in her left arm, nor could she close her hand. At the end of her annual exam, I asked her if she would like to try some new BodyTalk procedures that I learned to do. She responded favorably. We did just what is called the essential general treatment of balancing the system. Afterward, she sat up on the exam table and said, 'I guess something happened.' The next week she came in and all the feeling had come back into her left arm; everything felt completely normal."

"Now, not everybody responds this way. It [BodyTalk] clearly is not effective with everybody. However, about 70% of patients have incredible results. And, not all people would be open to engaging in the treatment. It's something out of the ordinary, not what you would expect from a physician. But, it's amazing the things that you get exposed to when you start on this path."

The Healing Arts Center also has become a central educational resource. On the expanding list of treatment therapies is Family Constellation Dynamics Therapy. In his book, *Love's Hidden Symmetry*, Bert Hellinger suggests a generational link between certain circumstances and experiences that happen within the family.[7] Without intervention, they are likely to be repeated in subsequent generations. There are important consequences of such links to both physical and emotional health. When the center opened, Lon invited Victoria Schnable from Freiburg, Germany, to conduct a family matrix workshop. Although her worldwide teaching schedule is usually booked 2 to 3 years in advance, she accepted. Out of the initial workshop grew a 1½ year training program for people to do Family Constellation Therapy.

Describing himself as a bit of a maverick, Lon appears clear in his understanding of what it takes to be a good physician. He states, "First and foremost is the relationship the physician has with the patient, although I hesitate to use the word 'patient' because it can relegate a person to an inferior role. Whatever the word, the doctor and the person being served are on a journey together. I think a lot of what we do is not just medical; the relationship can be therapeutic for both of us. Somehow the relationship heals as much as the diagnosis and treatment."

Of course, there must be technical competence, but Lon cautions against treating patients as a technically competent mechanic might change the oil in an automobile. And, he includes another factor. "To be a good doctor," he states, "there needs to be the joy of doing medicine. I know so many docs who are very

[7] Hellinger B. *Love's Hidden Symmetry*. Phoenix, AR: Zeig, Tucker & Co; 1998.

depressed and very unhappy. But for me, an authentic doctor is a person who is immersed in the joy of living. This doesn't mean we can't be sad or depressed at times. But we need to be authentic in each moment. I think it's hard for a lot of docs to be authentic because people tend to put us on a pedestal, not wanting to see the non-doctor side of our personalities. So some doctors go through life revealing only one side of themselves."

Lon also views healing in a more holistic sense, helping people along their journey in life, and it doesn't necessarily just mean physical or mental healing. He explains, "Healing can be very painful and tragic. It involves submitting to a person's destiny and allowing that person to become peaceful with it."

"If a person has a disease, I think that a lot of people identify themselves with it. In identifying with a disease, they become that disease. That is very dangerous because people walk around saying, 'I'm diabetic' or 'I'm arthritic.' Healing sometimes takes place when they start to differentiate themselves from an ongoing disease. It is more appropriate to say, 'I am a person and there is diabetes, or there is arthritis.' Once you differentiate in this manner, healing can be more effective. Otherwise, in a sense, if you kill the disease, you kill the person. It's an interesting difference to say, 'This is a problem; I am not my problem,' just as you might say, 'This is my father; I am not my father.' Technically, this is called disassociation or not labeling oneself, thus preserving a sense of individuality. Again, it can contribute to the healing process."

"Sometimes the ultimate healing for a person is in death. So, for me there is nothing frightening about death. Obviously, death is as common as birth, so we need to accept it as part of reality and not deny it."

Lon recalls one patient who illustrates his point. "I had a patient for years, a wonderful gal who had breast cancer and who chose not to do anything conventional in Western medicine about it. We did some things that allowed her to recapture her life again. She had been a person who was really not in charge of her life, living in a dysfunctional family. She cleaned up her diet, started to exercise, and for a year and a half she became extremely healthy. She assumed a stance in life that she had never had access to before. She became extremely successful in real estate and was immensely happy. I continued to see her through this whole process. Finally, she decided that her relationship with her husband was not healthy and she needed to leave him, which she did. Then within about a week she developed a new lump and very rapidly her health went downhill."

"We might ask, once she had finally regained her own self sense of power and femininity, no longer willing to be abused physically and mentally, why would she get worse? We talked about it, and her response was that now she felt complete. She didn't need to stay here anymore. She'd finally done her last act of reclaiming her power and she didn't need to do these other things anymore. She had become herself and was complete. She died about 3 weeks later, a very, very contented person."

"We tend to think of stories as being successful if we defeat the enemy of disease. But disease isn't the enemy," he says emphatically. "It's a teacher. So the question goes back to what are we doing as physicians? What is healing? What is this all about? And I don't think we know."

Lon's insights square with some of the perceptions of quantum physicists. We live in a universe containing many dimensions, a multiverse and not a universe. Some also claim that time is circular as well as linear, so apart from a person's particular faith or belief system, we have no idea about what occurs after death.

Such a perception can take the sting out of death and allow us to lighten life with humor and optimism. Humor serves as an important element in Lon's practice. "There is always laughter in each day," he says. "We get together each Thursday morning as a staff and there is lots of laughter." Although he does not specifically link his appreciation of humor to his view of the future of medicine, one suspects that there is a relationship. Optimistic and hopeful about the future, Lon affirms, "The profession continues to evolve and change. If you can't recognize and accept this, then you can get stuck in a kind of perpetual past. So I'm all for human nature that for thousands of years has been able to change and grow. Although tragedy obviously exists as a part of the life cycle, I see a world that is generally good. If you can't celebrate the whole thing, then I guess you get stuck in being cynical and judgmental."

Agreeing that some people are going to leave medicine, he states, "I think some doctors are making judgments like the way they make diagnoses; here we have an illness that must be cured. I don't see it that way at all. For example, I view managed care as a learning experience and a fantastic experiment. In general, I believe people initiate change with an intent to do good."

Laughing and exaggerating to make his point, he says, "I don't see people attempting to say, 'Well, let's develop a new way to make a lot of money in medicine. Let's manipulate people into having bypass surgery so we can prevent them from learning how to eat right, change things, and keep them sick.' There may be some big businesses and some pharmaceutical companies that potentially can do some things that feel threatening. But, if you get caught up in that belief, you can't be effective as a doctor."

We asked Lon about his heroes. There is no one particular hero to whom he looks for inspiration. Rather, he credits many people with influencing his life. "I think that there are lots of people in life who were absolutely gifts to me. I incorporate their insights into my personal journey."

A quote currently hanging on his wall best personifies his belief. It reads, "What's going to happen is not in your hands. So forget about what is going to happen and do your duty." Laughing, he says, "I just love it. It has a healthy disrespect for thinking that we are responsible for outcomes. I think that's one of the problems we have in medicine; we are so serious about results."

Lon sees his practice as a spiritual journey. "I don't use terms such as *spirit* or *soul* unless others use them. I don't want to box them into that. I am very comfortable with people wherever they are and am nonjudgmental about the decisions they made to get them to where they are."

Referring to another of Bert Hellinger's books, *Acknowledging What Is*,[8] he explains, "The book represents a nice set of liturgies about family constellations and philosophy of life." Having read the book, we believe that Family Constellation Dynamics Therapy is based, at least in part, on the perceptions presented in the introduction to this book, namely, that the universe is essentially a weblike field of energy where everything is connected or constellated. Everything belongs! So, in terms of a family system, a tragedy may occur, such as a divorce or a death caused by perhaps a suicide. Suddenly, the family system becomes psychologically unbalanced and remains this way even though one person may be physically removed or dead. People remain entangled in the event until the constellation is brought out in the open and addressed. Then, understanding, acceptance, and healing can

---

[8] Hellinger B. *Acknowledging What Is*. Phoenix, AZ: Zeig, Tucker & Theisen; 1999.

occur. It's quite compatible with the concept that "you shall know the truth, and the truth will set you free."

Concluding, Lon affirms, "Family Constellation Dynamics Therapy is extremely nonjudgmental. All of a sudden, when you start to recognize the dynamics of how people get to where they are, the history beliefs and behaviors passed from generation to generation, you become very accepting of them. If patients wish, I symbolically walk with them for awhile and it is an honor to be able to do that."

TEACHERS/MANAGERS

"Medicine men aren't horses. You don't breed them."
—Lame Deer
Sioux Medicine Man

Servant Scientist

Douglas S. Paauw, MD

In some ways, Dr Doug Paauw's circuitous route to medicine might be best described as one of kicking and protesting. As he tells the story, looking through the rearview mirror of his life to his mother's wisdom, he did not intend to become a physician.

"I had a fairly unusual pathway to becoming a doctor," he remembers. "I knew early in life that I wanted a career where I could work with and help people. In this respect, for some reason, my mother felt that the best career would be in medicine. At the time, because she believed it was a good idea, I took the opposite pole and thought it would be a bad choice," he says smiling. "I rebelled to the point of moving as far away from medicine as possible by becoming a Christian Scientist. I wasn't conscious of this rebellion at the time, but what I learned from the experience was that some people could live very healthy lives without medication or having an MRI scan. These are tools that can help us when a person is in a diseased state, but they do not represent the core of what health is all about. I learned that people can live long, healthy lives and when there is illness, healing can occur without the technology."

"We need to understand this," Doug continues, "because one of the dangers of medicine is the possibility of actually hurting people. Doctors can recommend and engage in treatments that actually make people sicker than when they first came in for a visit. Without a healthy respect for this possibility, you might end up harming more people than you help."

"This is a rather long-winded way of getting to the issue of career choice," he says, "but when I finished college I realized I was avoiding the field of medicine. When I finally combined my interests in science and service, I realized I could make a big difference by taking care of people. Frequently you will hear medical students telling you that they had an inspirational doctor when they were young whom they viewed as a role model. For me, it was the opposite; the role models were negative. I was exposed to health care providers who didn't listen and communicate very well. Instead, being busy, they lacked the ability to hear what my family or I had to say. So if I planned to become a doctor, I wanted to engage in a different kind of practice."

In college, he majored in biology and minored in chemistry, disciplines that were not incompatible with Christian Science. His interests in water, fish, and fish life cycles served as a hobby and as a potential career. However, he soon realized that he would be unhappy simply working with ecosystems and not with people.

He declared, "My fundamental passion involves exploring the question of why healthy people become sick. What changes occurred in their lives that may have contributed to the illness? How quickly did they realize they were sick? How did the illness impact their functioning and their families?" It was around this time that he left the Christian Science religion.

"From the day I began medical school, I never regretted the decision or looked backward. I loved the experience, including the first 2 years when we were in class for 40 hours each week. On top of this, I had to study another 40 to 60 hours to learn all of the material. I never was bothered by it because I enjoyed the subjects. I also loved teaching and spending a lot of time with my classmates. Many students can't wait to get the first 2 years behind them, but I was thrilled with them."

There is no question that today medicine is Doug's passion. For him, passion involves waking up every day excited about going to work.

"My work as a physician is much more than a job or a career," he emphasizes. "I never separate my role as a doctor from my personality, as though you would put on a different persona after you left the office. I enjoy having my patients and their needs in my thoughts during working hours and even thereafter. We doctors have an opportunity to care about people's lives in a rather unique way. I live for the moments when I can make a difference in human caring both through healing and also by listening to their stories."

Doug believes that effective medicine involves a combination of listening and responding with wisdom. It involves the use of both patience and common sense. Obviously it includes having a very broad understanding of the science of medicine, but without other more humanly interactive skills, becoming a good physician is very difficult. Does the patient articulate a clear understanding of his/her goals? If not, a good physician can help to clarify them. Is the patient seen as a compilation of medical problems, or as a whole person with a life history, emotions, aspirations, and spiritual needs?

Doug believes that much of the healing process is not associated with tests and medication. "Sometimes they can actually get in the way of healing," he states. "Of course, most often they are crucial to the process, but without a plan and someone to talk to about concerns, frustrations, and fears, what a physician can accomplish is very much muted. Listening and being able to communicate make all the difference in having a helpful role in people's health. Sometimes by listening, you discover that the best thing to do is help a person accept the problem, as opposed to conducting additional tests or increasing medications. We can actually cause more sickness physically and mentally through the application of technology. Three different people coming to the office with the same disease may end up with three different treatment plans based on who they are and on their needs."

Doug understood the importance of listening to his patients early in his training. He thoroughly enjoyed his clerkship because it afforded him the opportunity of hearing people's stories.

"As a medical student, you have fewer patients, so you have more time to spend with them," he recalls. "Great personal reward came from spending an hour or two with each of them, explaining their disease, and meeting with their families. The stories that I heard from patients were incredible. For example, on a high-risk OB clerkship, I remember talking to one woman, 24 weeks pregnant, whose baby was stillborn. During a counseling session afterward, she told me that she needed to go to the grocery store before returning home. She said she had to do this in order to bring something back into the house. At the time, it struck me about the many ways people deal with loss and grief. For her, it was important to walk into the door of her home with her arms full of something."

Doug continues, "I remember a patient I had who taught me so much about living and who gave me a message that I have carried with me to this day. She was a wonderful, 63-year-old woman whose husband was approaching retirement age and who adored her three grandchildren. She entered the hospital because of terrible back pain. Her neighbor, who was a medical professor, directly admitted her without any previous examination because he knew how much she was suffering. After an initial examination, I realized that she might have a tumor and ordered tests which confirmed the existence of cancer that had spread throughout her body."

"I remember being the one having to announce the bad news. I had spent about 4 hours with her up until this time and felt really connected to her and the family. It was the first time I had ever had to break the news of a fatal illness. They listened to me and I was able to provide some comfort. She was in the hospital for about a week, waiting for more tests, and every day I spent an hour or so with this woman listening to her story and about the people in her life. She and her husband also took great interest in my career, where I was going for my residency, and what my goals were for the future. Here were incredible people facing death with a genuine concern for me!"

"The last day I visited her in the hospital, she gave me a card with a 50-dollar bill in it. Shocked, I thought about the ethical implications. However, the card said that they wanted me to take my wife out to dinner. They said that I had given up so much of my time to be with them instead of my wife. They hoped that we would enjoy each minute of our lives because we never know when it will end. I remember this lady almost every day and when I counsel patients about chronic diseases that are not fatal, I let them know that they have choices in terms of how to cope with their problems and how they still can contribute to the quality of their lives. So, the messages I receive along the way from my patients help me to formulate what I do as a doctor."

There are many such stories in Doug's medical career, and he acknowledges that his patients have taught him about life and death. In many ways their relationship has been a gift. One such gift has made a profound difference in Doug's life long after his patient's death. One Indonesian patient brought with her a box of Chinese pastry during every visit. She had kidney failure and had to come in every other week. Chuckling, he says, "One day, she was having greater difficulty and I was going to have to see her fairly soon, so we squeezed her into the schedule on a Monday morning at 10:00 rather than the usual Wednesday afternoon. There was a big commotion at the front desk. They told me that the woman absolutely refused to come at 10 am. She told us that she could not come at this time because the Chinese bakery doesn't open until 11 am."

This woman, her family, and Doug grew very close over this period of time. She eventually died, and he helped in the timing of her death by turning off her ventilator according to her custom. Her family has adopted Doug and his family into their family and today the two families share special dinners and activities. Their continuing friendship has been an enriching gift for all of the Paauws'.

Today, Doug is an associate professor of medicine at the University of Washington School of Medicine and is the faculty advisor for internal medicine students. In his position, it is easy to contrast his own medical training with today's education.

He recalls only one unpleasant experience as a student. During his OB rotation, he was taking care of patients in the wards. A woman had a fever and was coughing up blood. "It was clear to me," he observed, "that she was having a blood clot in her lungs. I put her on oxygen and scheduled her for a test to confirm my diagnosis. I was proud of myself, but a resident doctor yelled at me very loudly, announcing that I was the stupidest medical student she had ever seen. She was angry that I had not initiated a standard 'fever workup.' She could have taken me aside and counseled me, but instead yelled at me in front of a number of other people. However, this was the only time during my training that I was mistreated."

Doug suggests that it is a very different environment today. While he had one day off each month during his training, today he oversees a program where students have 5 or 6 days off each month. They may still work 70 hours a week, but they don't work the 100-hour weeks typical in earlier times. Also, he says, training seems a lot more abusive if you don't like what you are doing. For example, some of us would consider working 40 hours a week packing bags at a grocery store to be vocational abuse.

As with most physicians, Doug has had to cope with mistakes and setbacks in his practice. "I always tell my students that for every time we look like we know what we are doing, it's because we've learned from other people's mistakes," he says. "Hopefully, this remains in the forefront of our consciousness and we won't make the same mistake twice."

"I remember when I was an intern taking care of a very nice 70-year-old man with a heart murmur. With very little supervision at the time, I diagnosed the murmur and sent him for a treadmill test to see if he had a bad angina, and also for an echocardiogram. He passed the tests, but then developed very atypical symptoms of heart failure. I treated him and he improved. But, about a month later, he simply dropped dead at home. I felt very guilty, because it suddenly dawned on me that we should have replaced a heart valve. I constantly dwelled upon the reality that I didn't have enough knowledge to know what to do and that he might have been alive today if I acted differently. He had multiple problems such as diabetes, so he might have died from other causes. But I carried the guilt and feeling of being inadequate for a long time. Today, when teaching medical students, I remind them how important it is to act appropriately and quickly in certain situations. We should know the things that, if we do not do them, a person may die. But, nonetheless, doctors make mistakes because they are human. If you cannot accept this reality, you can't be a doctor."

"Shown our mistakes and forgiven them, we can grow, perhaps in some small way become better people. Mistakes understood in this way are a process, a way to connect with one another and with our deepest selves."

— David Hilfiker, MD
Healing the Wounds (1985)

Continuing, Doug affirms, "Everyone dies, but we can make a big difference in people's lives, making diagnoses that save lives. However, we may also miss opportunities. I've become more philosophical, thinking that over the course of a number of years I may have saved 10 lives, but could possibly have saved 17 of them. But," he cautions, "you can't get down on yourself for not being perfect. The trick is not getting too high about your successes or too low about the failures."

What Doug hopes is that when it's all said and done at the conclusion of his life, he wants his patients to remember him by saying, "that I listened and cared about them. Also, that I was honest with them and that they never had a better doctor."

Doug loves to share some of the more humorous antidotes associated with his practice. "There are so many funny things that have happened to me that make great stories," he reports. "I have a whole group of patients with whom I share jokes. Depending upon the person, I even share the so-called dirty jokes. For example, when I was in a family practice rotation in medical school, I counseled a woman who came in for her annual physical. I asked her if she was using birth control. She assured me that they were and said that her husband used condiments. Laughingly, I told her that I suppose they might work."

Doug says he can't think of a day when he doesn't laugh with his patients. "One of my more recent funny stories comes from being in a high technology university setting. We had a patient coming in for a complete physical exam by one of our residents. The resident did all of the screening appropriate for a 55-year-old woman. But she said, 'I know you are doing all of these things, but I really want to have the new specialized test for colon cancer. I want the digitized rectal exam.' Now, what is called a digital rectal exam is simply putting a finger in someone's bottom and feeling for a lump. She had come a long way to get the new, specialized test, figuring that the university would have the most modern equipment! The resident had to explain that the modern equipment was on the end of his hand."

More soberly, Doug shares his reflections on the current changing health care environment. He believes that human interaction must be present in the profession. He recently attended a presentation by a computer technologist who suggested that in the future we would be introduced to virtual medicine, where the physician is in his office and the patient is at home. Both sit in front of their computers for a short 4-minute transaction. Doug finds such predictions worrisome and expresses his concern over the lack of opportunity for laying on of hands or physical examination.

"The problem with any type of virtual interaction is that things are not the same over the phone or on the computer. Can you imagine breaking negative news to someone over the computer, whether it is a physical problem or a depression? You have to look at a patient and speak empathetically, helping them to understand their situation. The human side of medicine will never be replaced, because people need to talk to people."

Doug trusts that current trends will not continue limiting human contact with physicians and the necessity of contacting insurance companies for every medication a patient might require. He fears that today, cutting costs is often of greater value than the quality time spent with the patient. He knows of several instances where physicians have given up their practices because of having to work 80 hours a week just to have a reasonable income. However, he is convinced that if both patients and physicians value human contact, then eventually it will change.

Doug acknowledges the importance of the less tangible aspects of medicine, such as spirituality and prayer. He believes that people must really see themselves as one entity in order to heal. He declares, "We can treat people with medication, but they must have a sense of wholeness, including a spiritual identity. To some degree, this reflects my experience with Christian Science. Their perspective on spiritual healing hinges on the belief that we are created in the image and likeness of God. Mistakes, problems, and accepting limitations cause illness. So their approach is not to dwell on a disease such as cancer or diabetes, but to get back to the notion of being created in the image of God."

"In any case," he continues, "my previous exposure to this perspective has helped me to view people not simply as a compilation of diseases. Also, I believe prayer is very important and I pray for my patients. I tell them when appropriate that I include them in my prayers. Of course, we don't always know where a person stands on such matters. But, regardless of where a patient stands with respect to religion or spirituality, I have yet to have a patient ever seem the least bit offended. They are often very touched by it, as though you are doing something very powerful for them. I believe it has something to do with a doctor recognizing that he or she does not have all the answers. Of course, we must use good judgment."

In addition, he declares, "I think the power of healing resides in part in a person's belief system. I don't think it's necessarily mind over matter, as though we could will ourselves to health. Rather, it's the ability to believe that one's body can get better and that you can function even with limitations. This can even impact more critical problems. In medicine, we certainly do witness miracles. We experience people surviving well beyond anything that could be explained medically."

With considerable emotion, Doug recalls the following story. "This is a tear-jerking story, but I had a patient who was diagnosed with lung cancer in 1982, and the cancer had spread around her heart. Usually the prognosis for this is death within a month. She received therapy and her cancer went into remission; they could not find it anymore. Thereafter, she received no further treatment and had no evidence of disease for about 10 years."

"Then, she came to me again with severe pain, and we discovered a cancer in her lung that eroded into her arm. Any motion of her arm resulted in terrible pain. She eventually went to a hospice, where I visited her. She spoke about the realization that she would not be alive much longer, but really appreciated the 10 years, which she viewed as a gift. She died about a week later."

"Then, about 3 months after her death, I received a call from her daughter, asking for a visit with me. She worked at our hospital and I knew her fairly well. She brought a bag with her and out of it she pulled a beautiful, hand-stitched quilt. Each patch contained a picture of a little girl with a parasol. My patient knew that I had a young daughter and, despite the terrible pain in her arm, she had been making this quilt for me to show her appreciation. She had died with three little squares left undone. And so, her daughter took a quilting class so she could finish her mother's gift. For me, the thought of someone putting up with so much pain in order to express his or her gratitude, well, I just could not stop crying. But, for many of us [doctors], our careers are filled with stories like this one."

Hitting a Home Run

Marc Demers, MD

Surgical oncologist, Dr Marc Demers, tells us enthusiastically, "I think I've hit a home run professionally; I couldn't be happier." Although Marc displayed an interest in medicine earlier, his first exposure to it began when he was 14 years old.

"A friend of my father was an anesthesiologist at a local hospital," he recalls. "He knew I was interested in being a doctor and took me into the operating room. I saw some surgery that became life changing. A light went on, seeing the excitement in the operating room and the things that surgeons could do. It impressed me almost like nothing else. I still carry an image of that day. It happened before you could watch an operation on television. In those days medicine and surgery were cloaked in a lot more secrecy than today."

"However, " Marc confesses, "as you mature in surgery the excitement begins to fade somewhat. But, I find oncology to be incredibly important, an opportunity to bring order to chaos. It is fascinating in many different ways and quite satisfying."

Marc has been in medicine almost 9 years. Originally from the Boston area, he went to medical school at Boston University and later did his oncology residency at M. D. Anderson in Houston. He began his career in academic medicine at Case Western in Missouri. Today, he is part of a surgical group practice in the Orlando area. Explaining his movement from academic medicine to a clinical practice, he says, "I have a clinical practice that includes training interns at a regional hospital. I made the shift because it was a unique opportunity to go into practice with a long-time friend who has since died."

Marc believes the heart of medicine touches the nature of soul. "When you strip away medical practice from the things that are necessary, the fact that we have to make a living, manage an office, and maintain a relationship with a hospital—strip that away and it comes down to patient care. That is the center of why we practice medicine."

Continuing he says, "I think that's what drives us to medicine, what attracted us to it in our formative years. It's hard to put your finger on it. It has to do with performing in difficult situations where actions really matter; making an important contribution to people's lives when they are vulnerable and have need. That's basic!"

Continuing, Marc exclaims, "Medicine is my passion. Career choices often stem from urges within your psyche that you may be unconscious of. For me, one thing clear is that I need a profession that is tangible, clearly important to people with results reinforced every day. It would be difficult for me to be a theoretical physicist for a number of reasons, but especially because I could not be certain about making a tangible contribution. Going home everyday after doing surgery, I have no question that I made a contribution that day."

Marc believes passion means having an attachment for and a love of what you do. "It goes beyond just having a job, but sometimes calls forth heroic energies." With passion, income or status or other things we generally think about as rewards don't drive you. It drives you for its own reasons. I don't think you can shake it."

Marc views medicine as a calling. "To be honest, if I couldn't be a surgeon, I probably wouldn't be in medicine. Surgery is unique. It's very different from being another kind of doctor." Marc states that, if tomorrow he could no longer practice surgery, he knows he would find another way to make a living, but nothing else would satisfy that passion.

For lay people, a surgeon is often considered the personal instrumental in correcting a physical problem. We wondered how Marc sees healing. He does not believe healing is synonymous with cure.

"They are totally different things. Surgery is very much the nuts and bolts of the job and if you don't attend to the very physical part of surgery, you're not a really great surgeon. So, healing has to mean some very basic things to a surgeon that it may not mean to a counselor or someone who deals with other aspects of it. Tissues come together and body parts begin to work normally again, returning them to a premorbid state."

Again, he emphasizes, "We don't always heal and we certainly don't always cure. Anything we would consider doing with a patient wouldn't be done if we anticipated healing wouldn't happen. Everything is done with the idea toward healing but it doesn't always happen."

Marc also believes the power to heal is related to some kind of biological reserve, although some people may have a greater reserve than others. Amplifying, he explains, "Teenagers usually heal faster than 80-year-olds. You can do the same operation to a number of different people, all of whom, relatively speaking, may have the same biology, but the ability to heal and return to normal are impacted in large measure by their own notion of themselves. Do they view themselves as chronically ill persons? If they do, they will be chronically ill. If they see themselves as an incredibly vigorous person, who can overcome huge obstacles, chances are pretty good that will occur. If they see themselves as someone who will probably never be able to go back to work and are expecting to be disabled, they will probably be disabled."

Marc believes in a strong relationship between prayer, spirituality, and healing. "I have a very strong notion about the need to pray; both for me and for my patients. For me, I need to pray because what I do doesn't always work. And, every time you perform a difficult surgery, you run the risk of harming someone, causing an injury from which they may not be able to recover. As much as it's easy to take credit when something goes very well, it's personally devastating when something runs afoul despite your best efforts. So I think you have to remind yourself there are larger forces at play in the outcome of things in our lives. This humility comes with prayer and becomes vital to going on with my job. I usually pray before surgery, especially the big ones. I don't ask for much when I pray. I do ask that my talents be used as best they possibly can be on behalf of the patient."

While patients might ask him to pray for them, more often than not, he explains, patients offer to pray for him. "I love when they ask. I think that's great." He notes that the subject comes up about once a day in the office. "A lot of patients are very up front about their spirituality, much more so than I am in general. I have patients who, before operating on them, routinely tell me they will pray. Many surgeons pray more frequently than you might think."

As Marc noted earlier, when things don't go well, it can be devastating. We asked him how he personally handles such disappointments and how medical students might be counseled about failures. "I had a patient with stomach cancer," Marc remembers. "He was about 40, vigorous looking, but about 7 days after surgery he died. You have to deal with it on a number of levels. You have to deal with the anger of the family directed toward you because you were involved in the event. You have to deal with it personally, asking what you did or not do that might have led to a bad outcome. And, you have to deal with the fact that you had someone walk into your office who came under your care and who died. That is irrevocable and final," he emphasizes.

"In our system, the way we train residents is through weekly morbidity and mortality conferences, where all complications and deaths are presented to all the surgeons who attend that hospital. It can be uncomfortable, but it's a very healthy approach. I suppose it could be embarrassing for some people, but in the light of day everyone looks at the same information and you can be absolved of some of the responsibility. The conference is difficult, but it shows the limits of what you can do."

With regard to a medical student's first experience of a mistake, he remarks, "How do you prepare someone to ride a bike? The first time you ride, you fall. I don't know how you cushion the blow. There is a great phrase having to do with surgical training from the book, *Forgive and Remember*," he tells us laughingly. "'Everything we do to harm someone in surgery, by all means we will forgive you. But, we will remember it and so will you. Don't repeat it. Try to better yourself.'"

In fact, Marc believes one of the primary characteristics of a good surgeon has to do with being honest with oneself, about what you can and can't do. "Only if you have humility about your abilities can you be honest in your appraisal of what you can and can't do for somebody," he says. "Actually, humility and honesty represent two sides of the same coin."

Another important characteristic is perseverance. "After a bad experience, I still have to get up the next day and do it again. If I perform a big operation on someone and they die, that afternoon I may have to put somebody through the same surgery. You must be able to perform repeatedly under circumstances that are less than optimal. You may be exhausted but still have to give your very best. Perseverance even trumps brilliance. Finally," he says, "a good surgeon must use judgment, always recognizing what is and what is not possible."

Over the course of his practice, Marc experienced amazing patient outcomes in situations that shouldn't have gone well. "When I was in my fellowship at M. D. Anderson, we saw all kinds of patients with advanced cancers. We operated on many cancers knowing they would reoccur. Often patients with stomach cancer die from it. Typically the vast majority of patients having stomach cancer that is metastatic to surrounding lymph nodes will die within a year or two."

"However, I will never forget a little Hispanic lady who came in after a total gastrectomy, with the surrounding cancerous lymph nodes removed. Thirteen years later she returned for her annual checkup!" he declares. "It is almost unheard of for someone to live with that kind of tumor burden. For me, that was the first unexpected great outcome from cancer. It impacted me because I had never seen it before."

"So, what can you say to someone with such advanced disease? We tell them that we just don't know all the factors that go into curing, the way the hand of God works. Sometimes you do see remarkable things."

Marc suggests that young people contemplating medicine or surgery as a career should first be exposed to the field. "I think someone who is committed to medicine as a career will not become discouraged. I think if you get significantly discouraged, then by all means choose something else. Those who firmly believe it's the right thing won't be discouraged by someone suggesting it as a poor career choice; it won't be enough to keep them away."

He adds, "Surgery is almost like a baptism by fire, and the attrition rate is high. About a third of those starting their surgical residencies never finish. It's 5 years of chronic fatigue, lack of sleep, lost social life, being away from your family, working for peanuts. There is very little reward but the work itself. It's a difficult and long period in one's life."

To those who may argue that medical school is abusive, Marc neither agrees nor disagrees, saying, "I don't think the answer comes easily. There are certainly abusive elements of medical school and residency training going far beyond what you do in almost any other job, save the military. I can't think of another type of employment that requires the kind of exhausting work that we do. That may feel abusive to some people. Working with some surgeons can be very difficult. Undoubtedly some abusive people in medical education enjoy having younger, bright people under their thumb. But in the main, I don't believe it is offensive."

Marc agrees that being female might affect their treatment in the field. "I think being a female makes a difference. It is more difficult for a woman in some ways and in some ways easier.

Educators may show greater difference to women trainees. Personally," he admits, "around women, my language gets cleaned up. I am a little more polite. I think it's difficult whenever a man or woman goes into a field dominated by the other gender."

Marc particularly loves training residents. "I have never worked in a situation where I didn't have them around me. Personally, I was treated well as a resident. When I look back at the way people trained me, I am nothing but grateful. I was tired, certainly worked to exhaustion, but I never felt that those who trained me had anything but my best interests and the interests of the patients at heart. I hope I am treating my residents the same way."

"If they taught me nothing else, the surgeons taught me that delivering high-quality humane care is hard work."

— Charles L. Bosk
Forgive and Remember (1979)

Reflecting on the changing, sometimes chaotic, health care environment, Marc is decidedly optimistic about medicine, although he agrees the climate is more difficult today. "However, surgery is a unique field," he states enthusiastically. "You get to do things that no one else gets to do. So, in this respect, I'm always optimistic. Administrative overload is always incredibly frustrating and infuriating and we complain often, but such issues are not at the center of our practices. Medicine and surgery stand at the center, an incredible way to spend your days. As a surgeon, every day you have an opportunity to see new things that you have never seen before. It's like seeing a great sunset! You see a particular condition being displayed in a way that is new. You see the inner workings of the human body on a daily basis. You witness wonder and the things that you can accomplish in the care of patients. What other job allows you to do that? I can't think of another job that allows you to do those things with such frequency."

Going With Grace

Richard Payne, MD

Having conducted more than 90 week-long retreats for cancer patients and their families, Rachel Naomi Remen, MD, declares, "For all these years, I have listened to people's stories, stories from the edge of life. These stories have changed me. They've inspired me. They've helped me to know what is important, what really matters. Dying people can teach us how to live well. Being with people who are dying is a refuge from everything that is not genuine in our culture. . . . Dying seems to be a process of dropping roles, of taking off masks, of stripping back to what might be called the Buddha seed, that birthright of integrity in all of us."[1]

Dr Richard Payne firmly agrees with Dr Remen, believing that stories serve as a powerful means of communicating. He sees them as ways for people to rethink how to view the world, change perspectives and actions. He believes this is especially true in his medical specialty, palliative care. He states, "In this field, at least currently, we see ourselves as operating on the fringes of medicine. We have a mission to make fundamental changes in the way medical care is provided to those facing the end of life."

Richard decided to enter the medical profession when he was a student in high school. An African-American, he grew up in a large family in Elizabeth, New Jersey. "One of the interesting things about growing up in the 1950s and 60s in cities like Elizabeth was that there was no de juror segregation, but it existed in a de facto sense," he declares. "Although we were quite poor, fortunately we happened to live down the street from some physicians, lawyers, and policemen. I got to know professional people on a fairly regular basis. I went to school with their children. In addition, I had an aptitude for the sciences and math, and was encouraged to be proficient in these studies."

Between his high school junior and senior years, he spent the summer in a National Science Foundation program in biochemistry. The subject greatly interested him, and because it was a national program, it helped him to develop a sense of competing

---

[1] Remen RN. *Final Wisdom* [audiotape]. Boulder, CO: Sounds True Recordings; 1998.

successfully with students from around the country. At this point,
it became clear that he wanted to be a physician. So after college,
he was accepted into Harvard Medical School, graduating in
1977. He did his internal medicine postgraduate training at Peter
Brigham Hospital in Boston, today called the Brigham and
Women's Hospital.

Richard's interest in neurology grew from his classes in the
neurosciences. "In medical school, I became interested in the neurosciences. You had to do at least 1-year internship in internal
medicine to qualify for a neurology residency. I went into medicine knowing I was headed in this direction. I thought about neu-
rosurgery, but reflecting back on it, I saw it as being a little too
militaristic for my taste. At least at a training level, it seemed
almost antiintellectual. I perceived that internal medicine and
neurology provided a little more freedom to disagree with the
professors," he smiles. He later completed a neurology residency
at the New York Hospital Cornell Medical Center.

We asked Richard whether as a young medical student he
experienced any discrimination. "I have to tell you," he responds,
"I was so driven to excel and be accepted in the best medical
school that I didn't perceive any discrimination. I'm sure it was
present and I remember some instances of racism in high school,
but I can't remember anything beyond that."

We asked Richard about what advice he might have for a student considering entering medicine. He answered, "I think that if
you are really interested in the medical profession, you should
pursue it. I believe there is a no more satisfying or noble career.
You always intend to do the right thing for people. Unfortunately,
you can't say this in every profession. There is no question that
you must work hard, but there is a tremendous sense of professional fulfillment."

There is concern today about the declining enrollment of
minority students in medical schools. Richard affirms this trend
and maintains that many public schools today, especially in urban
areas, are not providing students with the quality education
needed to enter medicine. In addition, he believes that there are
kids with the talent, but who get the message that unless you
have resources, medicine is beyond your capability. "Today, a kid
with my poor background (I was one of 13 children) might say
that it's out of his or her reach."

Like so many of the physicians we interviewed, Richard views medicine as a passion. Laughing, he says, "I don't see myself doing anything else in life other than perhaps being a sportscaster. I'm an old baseball player and could see myself in that arena. But, life is so short and so precious that the trick is to find what you really love and do it. I believe that our Creator gives each of us special talents; our task is to uncover and utilize them."

"I grew up in a very nurturing environment. My parents were not well educated, but they certainly knew the value of education. I also had a considerable amount of peer support. Unfortunately, the perception among many minorities today is that it's not cool to be smart. That drives me crazy."

Richard views passion as something you do that is all-consuming. It involves following a course of action that simply involves the right thing to do. "You can't hold back your enthusiasm," he says enthusiastically. (As Jim notes, enthusiasm is a word meaning "in God.")

His training prompted Richard to remain in academic medicine. In fact, he explains one of the reasons he went to Cornell's New York Hospital was, at the time, two of the most world-renowned neurologists were there. "Drs Fred Plum and Jerry Posner lead a strong academic program, training many of the current and future chairmen of neurology departments in the US. I went into palliative medicine as a by-product of this, because at Cornell, we spent time at the Memorial Sloan-Kettering Cancer Center. Early during my training I saw patients who had serious neurological complications caused by cancer, many of which were quite painful. I was exposed to role models, like Kathleen Foley, doctors with expertise in neurological assessment and in pain management. They were sensitive, caring, and very competent in their practices. They made a tremendous difference in the lives of their patients, even though a cure was impossible. This experience directed me to neuro-oncology and to pain management and palliative care."

Richard continues to have significant patient care responsibilities in addition to his teaching and research duties. As the chief of the Pain and Palliative Care Service at Memorial Sloan-Kettering Cancer Center, he supervises five other physicians, seven nurses, and a bereavement specialist. His research includes pharmacological studies of drugs used to treat pain and other symptoms. It also involves health service-related research, learning more about how to set up and deliver systems of care, especially to the medically underserved.

His responsibilities include a major training program, educating many of the leaders in pain management and palliative care in the United States. Every year they have four or five fellows in training, as well as students from other medical schools, coming from such faraway places as Australia and Korea.

Considering his intense work with cancer patients and pain medicine, we asked Richard to share some thoughts about the nature of healing.

"Healing works as a natural phenomenon that we can sometimes facilitate through medical and surgical endeavors and through assisting the patient with the ability to cope with an illness," he responds. "I believe that the patient has an active role in the process of healing. The power to heal resides within the biological and physiological systems of the body, but I'm open to the possibility and belief that we can influence these systems through psychological and physical processes. Also, things happen that promote healing that we certainly don't understand. We shouldn't be so close minded as to call it all magic."

Continuing, he says, "I do believe that healing is an important aspect of medicine, but not the only aspect. In many ways, this is the paradigm shift being discussed today with respect to palliative medicine. One can perform a legitimate function in medicine that doesn't necessarily involve complete healing or cure. It is taking us back to the ancient roots of medicine, when we could not cure and focused upon comforting patients."

Similarly, Richard believes that spirituality and prayer play an important role. Describing himself as both a spiritual and religious person, he says, "Prayer and spirit interact with the biological processes by promoting emotional well-being. This has effects in ways that I don't understand. I'm not sure I believe in divine intervention, but I know that prayer can make a difference. However, the scientist in me must ask how this can happen, and what I'm saying is that I don't know. My personal belief is that our Creator works through us. I've had patients who asked me to pray with them and I have done it. Or, I've sat in silence holding a hand while family members prayed. It seemed the right thing to do and I certainly felt better for having done so."

Calling on his experience, he says, "So often, patients who are dying, and their families in particular, ask why God doesn't or can't perform a miracle and cure this cancer. My response often is that I simply don't understand God's will. Personally, I've never had a patient with a chronically advanced disease within weeks of dying only to have a complete remission. I have heard of such stories and they have typically been with illnesses such as renal cell cancer and melanoma. With these, there can be interesting immunicological effects that can help arrest the disease."

> ". . . I have come to believe in something affirmed by every doctor who has found happiness in his work: that in the midst of death, we are in life."
>
> — David Loxterkamp, MD
> *The Measure of My Days*
> (1997)

In any case, today Richard is much more respectful and open-minded about attempting to understand the importance of a patient's psychological and emotional well-being. It plays an important role in healing and physical well-being.

He says, "As an intern or resident, I gave intellectual lip service to this, but today I am much more open to it. Also, I've grown in the sense of being much more willing to challenge the assumptions of the current health care system. I am more forcefully willing to advocate for the system to respect the wishes of patients, even if it causes inconvenience to customary practices. It's difficult because there is a lot of work to be done, but I am much more willing to fight the fight."

Sharing a very personal example of how medicine needs to return to more soulful roots, Richard tells us about his 84-year-old mother who faced advanced Alzheimer's Disease (and subsequently died). At the time of our interview, she just had been discharged from the hospital where she had a vascular surgical procedure.

"The surgeon who performed the procedure never really spoke to anyone in the family," he states. "Mom was very weak, had a very painful lesion in her foot, and couldn't walk, but the doctor was about to discharge her from the hospital. When asked about this by my sister who happened to be present during one of his rounds, he said, 'I thought she wasn't terribly mobile before the operation.' This remark made it very clear to my sister that he had not taken any time to get to know our mother. The fact was, until 3 weeks previously, she had been walking. I'm not suggesting that

he must be responsible for organizing all of the care required,"
Richard says emphatically, "but we've got to change the system
so that doctors are not simply technicians operating on a blood
vessel. Unfortunately, his behavior is becoming much more
common today."

Sadly, he declares, "My reaction was to get Mom out of that
environment, take her home, and take care of her, because I lost
confidence that anyone in that hospital system would treat her as
a human being. In fact, one of the huge attractions I have toward
palliative medicine is to humanize it. But I have to tell you that
we get people who rotate through our service complaining that
we spend too much time talking about patients' psychosocial
needs. They just want to know how to dose the morphine.
However, you've got to know who this person is and in a way,
you've got to integrate things at a level that is much more sophis-
ticated than simply having the technical skills."

Richard asserts that today, health care in general tends to see
itself as a series of problems to be solved. In one sense, he thinks
it is wonderful because we can treat so many illnesses successfully, but in another way it is a step backward. It reinforces a
lack of synthesis of care for the whole person. Today we face
superspecialization and intense pressure to get people into and
out of acute care settings. He asks, "Why expect things to
change in this kind of environment?" Answering his own question, he suggests, "Over time, and it may be a very long time,
the public will demand a more caring and humanistic approach
to health care."

We asked Richard about his colleagues' perceptions regarding
the current health care environment. He responds, "There are
many complaints, and I participate in the 'pity party' myself.
Most of the frustrations center around forced busy work, the
requirements for documentation, the need to justify treatments to
the third-party payers. I think that many doctors have romantic
memories of the old days, but the good old days weren't always
so good. Clearly, we have made tremendous medical advances; in
my practice, [as an example] there was much more physical suffering in the 'good old days.'"

As part of his teaching responsibilities, Richard talks to students about the softer skills of patient care, for example, how to
convey bad news to a patient.

"I sometimes worry about our ability to make a more enduring impact on young, prospective doctors," he says somewhat quietly. "This is why we need to address the subject in a very global and comprehensive manner. We need to educate not just medical students and residents, but practicing physicians and all hospital personnel. We need to address health policy on a very broad scope."

Richard involves himself in a number of organizations that seek to make such changes, such as the American Pain Society and the National Hospice and Palliative Care Organization. He serves on several advisory committees and federal panels. He declares, "Increasingly, I've been exercising my rights as a citizen by writing to legislators and becoming involved in political action to influence policy. This is part of our responsibility as citizens."

Richard has been a pioneer in bringing palliative care out of the dark ages. "In the late 1970s as I was finishing my training, I remember people telling me when I went on a job interview, not to mention the 'P' word, meaning palliation. People didn't want to hear about it, which is evidence of how much things have changed since then. I couldn't imagine hearing anyone saying that today. In fact, we can't produce enough doctors in the field; there are that many job opportunities."

"Back then it was appropriate to talk about the war against cancer and about pain management. The battlefield metaphors prevailed; there were winners and losers. Palliation was a gray area not for the winners."

"Also, one of the things I've gotten increasingly interested in is improving pain management care for the medically underserved, particularly the African-American community. The leaders of this community seem less interested in palliative care because they view the big picture as getting access to medical treatment. They are saying that if our people are dying from AIDS, cancer, and chronic renal failure, they don't want the system to tell them how to 'die better.' They want the system to eliminate the health care disparity. Palliative care in this context is misinterpreted, viewed as conflicting and placing attention on the wrong issue."

"So, one of my interesting challenges these days is going to bring the issue of palliative care out of the closet in the African-American community. Almost everyone will eventually need the care, and that's how it must be viewed. It doesn't mean that we should not also be promoting more access to curative treatment."

As we concluded our interview, Richard says he takes pride in the fact that he participates in a fringe group of hospice and palliative care that ultimately will make a significant difference in overall health care. "It's about getting back to the essence of medicine. As a child of the 1960s, I guess I have a rebellious mode. In 30 or so years, we may look back and identify hospice and palliative care as a movement that significantly helped to transform medicine. That would be nice!"

Healing Soul Mate

Janis D. Bridge, MD

D r Jan Bridge speaks of soul as the basic core values that we possess, the heart of a person's belief system. She says, "We are so busy all of the time, never having an opportunity to step back and reflect on such important matters as soul. Somehow the introspective part of our work gets lost. In terms of health care, soul refers to that mystery innate to a person and impacting well-being. Soul embraces our spirituality; it impacts our emotions. For example, I saw a patient this morning who is tuned in to interaction with other people and in a global sense to politics. My patient said that, after hearing Al Gore's concession speech, she cried deeply and became depressed, then developed a deep cough because she tends to internalize such events. So her soul is very much a part of her health perception. Anytime she becomes overly emotional, it impacts her physically."

For Jan, soul involves connecting with people, feeling like she is on the same wavelength with them. It does not mean that the outcome must be positive, but that she understands and empathizes with a patient. "Soul comes over you like a wave of warmth," she affirms. "You come out from a patient's room, and you feel that you are a brother or sister to that person. It doesn't happen that often, but there is some kind of love and warmth being generated."

"I remember one situation in particular in the hospital where I was attending to a woman with a very unfortunate cancer diagnosis. It left her with no hope at all for recovery; she was going to die in the hospital. But the connection between her, the family, and the hospital team members was awesome. The family asked a lot of questions about how to comfort the woman. We told them to do whatever made her feel better. We were not very specific, but it was a kind of human connection. It's fine to have a sense of your own soul, but unless your soul connects with another soul, it becomes less meaningful."

Jan's perspective is in line with what other people say about soul, and especially the perceptions of Thomas Moore in his book, *SoulMates*. Soul manifests itself in deep intimacy in specific places and with particular people. "A soulful connection can be found in families, on the job, in the neighborhood, with colleagues, and among friends, among longstanding acquaintances and in fleeting encounters, in socially sanctioned matings and in murky rendezvous."[2]

Specializing in internal medicine, Jan began her practice in 1994 at the age of 41. She also is an assistant professor of medicine at the University of Washington Medical School. Before entering medical school, she worked as a microbiologist and in public health in Los Angeles as an epidemiologist. During this period, she mothered two children and supported her husband as he studied to become a rabbi. She spent a year in Jerusalem during the first year of their marriage.

Jan decided to enter medicine because of her desire to connect with people. She always wanted to be a physician, but during her undergraduate years, she didn't believe she had the appropriate credentials. Microbiology became the next best thing because it was hospital-based, another way to work in health care. A fascinating study, it eventually led to an interest in infectious disease and epidemiology.

"I found myself interacting with public health nurses on outbreak investigations and the like. During these consultations, I became very envious of their ability to visit people's homes and relate directly with patients," she recalls. "Number crunching was my primary responsibility, whereas I discovered myself wanting to be the front-line caregiver. I told myself that I didn't want to be 65 and look back at my life regretting that I failed to follow my dream of being a doctor. My husband was supportive, so I decided to apply for medical school. I was lucky enough to be accepted and it's been a wonderful decision."

Jan perceives that entering medical school at a later age made it easier for her. "First of all," she states, "I was much better equipped to prioritize responsibilities in terms of spending time with my children and husband. I had to be very efficient in terms of study habits. Also, because of previous experiences, it was easier to learn and to interview patients during my rotations. Then too, I had some very supportive female friends in medical school, one who was actually older than me. Whenever faced with a dilemma or crisis, we would turn to each other for assistance. We continue to visit occasionally. Now our issues are different then in medical school, but we continue to support one another professionally and otherwise."

---

[2] Moore T. *SoulMates*. New York, NY: HarperCollinsPublishers; 1994: ix.

At the time she entered medical school, Jan had not determined a specialty, but knew she wanted to do something involving continuity of care because she especially enjoys developing relationships over time. She first thought about entering family medicine as opposed to internal medicine. However, during her clerkship, she discovered that working with older patients was most satisfying. She believes that older people have a lot on their plates to deal with in terms of having so many more life experiences.

"This is especially true with regard to adapting to loss," she notes. "They lose partners and friends, bodily functions, sometimes job status and loss of income. Growing older challenges us in so many ways. There is so much more to talk about in caring for older people." She found this path more rewarding than conducting well-child checkups.

"Passion," says Jan, "means that in my work, I never think about the clock. It's been this way from the beginning, when I first entered medical school. On Sunday evenings, some people talk about dreading the coming week. But for me, even when things are unsettling and stressful, I view each day as interesting and amazing. Every interaction with people is different; no day is the same in medicine."

Continuing, she says, "I talk to people in my profession who watch medical shows on television. While much of the drama is somewhat surrealistic, we all affirm that they do portray some of the daily excitement and diversity in medicine. You get to see what goes on behind the scenes. In the helping professions, you really have the opportunity to witness amazing things and make immediate connections. We hear deep secrets people reveal to few others. People often share what is going on in their lives in a very sacred way."

> "... in the privacy of the examining room, I was accorded the great privilege of talking about me, my feelings and aches and what's happening here and here and down here, and the doctor was not so bored to hear about it."
>
> — Garrison Keillor

"For example," she continues, "I had a patient whom I had seen for several years. About 4 or 5 years into our relationship, she told me her daughter confessed to being a lesbian. The mother asked me what I thought about that issue. At first, I didn't grasp what she was searching for, but she was Catholic and her question had a spiritual overtone to it. She really wanted to know whether being a lesbian was abnormal and wrong. Then, during the next visit she asked me if I believed in God and afterlife. She told me that she had always feared death. I thought to myself that it is an amazing thing to have such a conversation. She probably had these questions bottled up in her psyche for a long period of time. So, it makes me feel really good that people trust you enough to share such thoughts and concerns, even though you don't have all of the answers."

Jan believes it is vital to assess a person's spiritual orientation as well as his or her physical condition. And so, she sometimes initiates discussions about spiritual issues. She also sees a strong connection between spirituality and health, especially during times of deep stress. "When people face a serious illness with a negative prognosis, it's almost wrong if you don't explore their belief system," she states. "I help teach a spirituality-in-medicine course in a medical school. The thrust of this course is that a person's belief system can intimately impact health care."

"As a Jewish woman, I know that every Saturday in the synagogue a prayer is offered for those who are sick. In Judaism, one of the best deeds you can perform involves visiting a sick person. There is even a kind of folklore that if you visit such a person, you can take $\frac{1}{60}$th of their illness away. In fact, a protocol exists where you position yourself next to the bed, not standing above people but sitting at their level."

"A young man about my age attending our synagogue developed a serious lymphoma and went through a bone marrow transplant. During the high holy days, members of the congregation teamed up in his room conducting an all-day service that normally was held in the synagogue. The support of everyone was important to him and his family during the end of his life."

"I find that spirituality plays a significant role in how people process illness. Some people consider it to be a punishment from God for wrongdoing," Jan reveals. "I found this out once as a medical student doing a rotation in a rheumatology clinic. A young woman was recently diagnosed with rheumatoid arthritis. The endocrinologist said that the woman immediately began to cry during each visit. It was very early on in the illness, and only one joint was involved. She seemed to overreact. So I spoke to her for a while, attempting to bring her emotional reaction into the conversation. Eventually she informed me that she had an abortion when she was 15 years old. She said, 'I knew God would punish me some day.' So, someone like this woman definitely would benefit from further spiritual counseling."

Jan declines to identify healing with curing. She sees healing as somehow correlating with comforting. For her, the power to heal resides in the connection between the physician and the patient, but it is more in the mind of the patient than the physician.

"Two of the key, bridging tools involve listening and the laying on of hands," she states warmly. "Relative to touching, there are times when we don't examine a patient; they may come for a counseling visit. I have a number of patients who visit me for no physical reason, but for mental or emotional relief. However, I often touch them in an appropriate manner because they like it. Quite frankly, I guess they believe a doctor has more power then is actually the case. For example, when I touch them by listening to their heart, it may have a therapeutic benefit." Laughing and almost with tongue in cheek, she says, "They see you as some kind of authority with the power to heal."

This type of authority and power were discussed elsewhere in this book. The Swiss psychologist Carl Jung referred to the energy of the archetype of doctor. Used appropriately and even when the physician knows that she or he is human like the rest of us, it contributes to the healing process. When sickness enters the picture, slight, sometimes severe independence is lost; the patient might regress to childlike behavior. In *Power in the Helping Professions*, Adolf Guggenbühl-Craig states,

> "In such a situation the doctor becomes the great helper. He [she] is the source of all hope. Feared, respected, hated and admired, he [she] seems at times an almost godlike redeemer."[3]

Like refusing to appropriately administer an antibiotic, to dismiss such energy is to ignore a powerful source of healing. As in a parent–child relationship, to misuse it might equally cause harm and child abuse. In either case, it becomes vital to understand that such nonclinical power resides in the archetype more than in a physician's ego. We believe Jan radiates this kind of power and does so with great humility.

Relating healing to spirituality and prayer, Jan remarks that some of her patients have no interest in religion. "For others, healing and prayer remain quite connected. I had a mentally retarded patient, a young woman cared for in a family home. She developed a pancreatic tumor that was inoperable. When I gave

---

[3] Guggenbühl-Craig A. *Power in the Healing Professions*. Irving, TX: Spring Publications; 1979: 83.

the information to the caregiver, I had no hope to offer except that I would say a prayer for the young woman. I knew that the caregiver held spiritual beliefs, connected again to the Catholic Church. She seemed to appreciate my offer. It didn't heal the young woman, because she died. But, for many people we see on the oncology service, prayer is critical for them to cope with their illness and to feel some sense of hope. It's the hope that there is some guiding energy beyond us that can have an impact, something beyond the poisonous treatment of chemotherapy."

"Human love is not a substitution for spiritual love. It is an extension of it."

— Emmanuel

We asked Jan if she ever had an experience with a patient where she believed the outcome was going to be negative, yet for some reason a cure came about.

"Quite frankly, I don't really believe much in miracles," she exclaims. "However, I've seen situations defying conventional wisdom. I've been involved in situations, especially when supervising residents in the ward, when we are facing end-of-life situations. I always have an uneasy sensation about predicting death because, although it might appear eminent in a few days, you just never know."

"For example, a young man had an end-stage liver disease. It was so bad there was no hope for a transplant. His kidneys began to fail, and he had a very serious infection. By all conventional predictions he should have died, and I prepared the medical student to make sure we had his wishes in mind. We even had his family come from out of town to say good-bye. However, he rallied and turned around enough to leave the hospital. I don't consider it a miracle, but I also don't know what happened. Perhaps he was influenced by the arrival of his family whom he had not seen in a number of years because he had been in prison. The last I heard, he was doing fine."

Earlier in the interview, Jan stated that her husband was a rabbi, so we asked if and how his profession might connect with her practice of medicine. "My husband, Dan, visits a number of people in the hospital. He has a very comforting personality and bedside manner. When he visits someone we know personally, he holds their hand, brings his rabbi book, and offers a healing prayer; I see great power in these activities. People write beautiful cards about how much they appreciated his visits. So we have this connection, both of us caring for people who are ill, but in different ways."

"As director of the Jewish campus student center at the university, his congregation is made up of both students and faculty. And, since I teach, we are both connected to the university. Some of the Jewish medical students and residents participate in the center's worship and other activities."

"Finally, my husband engages in a considerable amount of student counseling, especially around issues of depression. I do the same with some of my patients. Sometimes we ask each other for advice, without breaking confidentiality or giving specific details. I find him to be quite knowledgeable and wise about many things. I believe he is proud of the fact that I am in medicine. In fact, when we first met, he wanted to be a doctor as well. Unfortunately, medical schools did not accept him and he faced a significant crisis about his career direction. After a few years, he put medicine to rest and decided to become a rabbi. I supported him through rabbinic school, and then he did the same for me during medical school. We have a lot invested in both careers. Our lives are hectic, but certainly not boring," she laughs.

Jan converted to Judaism just before she married 23 years earlier. Since she participated in both sides of the Judeo-Christian tradition, she understands both perspectives, although she claims she would be quite accepting even if she hadn't converted.

"Ever since I was 18 years old, I have been on a spiritual quest," she asserts. "I was brought up in the Congregational Church, but it didn't quite fit for me, so I explored the Quaker and the Sufi traditions. Then, during the 4 years I dated Dan, his family included me in all their rituals and practices. I received a good taste of what Judaism is all about."

Acknowledging that she has changed since entering medicine, she sees it as a natural progression. "I hate to say it, but I have become more realistic and less likely to become disappointed by people's behavior since graduation. I teach an introduction to clinical medicine group meeting almost once each week during lunch. I love it because it reminds me of what it was like when I first began school. I watch the videotape of their first interviews with patients," she smiles. "They are so eager and involved. Later on, however, you realize you can't help some people because they don't want to be helped. People are in charge of their own behavior. It simply became a natural realization for me over time."

Jan usually handles the grief she experiences in her practice by talking with her husband. She also visits with some of her colleagues who always make the time if she needs it. Reflecting upon her training, she suggests, "This is one of the pitfalls of residency training. You are so busy when on call on the wards. People die while you are gaining new patients. Someone you are connected with because you have cared for them dies and you never have a time to mourn. I tell students to at least take the time to speak with attending residents. This is especially vital if a mistake is made in treatment."

"We have a Day of Atonement in Judaism, when you fast and remain in the synagogue for most of the day. The idea is that you atone for your mistakes during the past year, asking for forgiveness from each person affected and from God. When the day is over you are sealed in the Book of Life for the next year."

She recounts one experience. "In the process of being deprived of food and introspecting on this, in one instance, suddenly all of the people in my practice who had died during the past year came into my consciousness. I was in tears and thought that I must have more grief to deal with than I was aware of."

We spoke to Jan about how she is handling the current health care system chaos. "Awhile ago I wasn't very resilient. I found myself buying into the belief that patients were products. There exists in medicine this issue of productivity, when for the sake of economics, standards are established in terms of the number of patients you are supposed to treat in a given day. I found this to be totally incongruent when caring for people. I found myself angry when people failed to show up, because I lost credit in terms of the numbers. However, eventually I realized that this was not why I entered medicine. I became a doctor to be present with people, so I gave up caring about productivity. I decided that it would play itself out one way or another. I make a reasonable effort to be productive, but I'm not going to fixate on it."

She states firmly, "My job is to listen to people and not set an agenda. Listening to patients is hard work and I often find myself fatigued. When I witness myself becoming short tempered with my patients or my family, then I know it's time to take a break and schedule a mini-vacation."

"Also, when I become upset about something in medicine, I am very vocal about it," she laughs. "Again, it's wonderful to have a support group of colleagues. My most recent tirade, and I'm thinking about writing an article about this, involves physician abandonment. It's the idea that health care coverage is tied to employment. I'll have a patient say to me that as of the first of the year, he or she cannot see me anymore because the insurance plan has been changed. It creates a great amount of anger on the part of both the doctor and the patient. It's like when you are young, out on a date, and someone dumps you. It feels like being marginalized. It undermines the soul of medicine."

Nonetheless, generally speaking, Jan remains optimistic about the future of health care. "I don't see how the system can survive in its present form. We find ourselves unable to do what people want from us, so eventually things will change. And, people are still applying to medical school in droves. It's a very special career, an amazing profession."

At the end of our interview, we asked Jan if she had a favorite poem or quote. Without hesitation, she points to a framed quotation of the Physicians Oath by Maimonides, a Jewish physician and philosopher who practiced in the twelfth century and who was called "The Prince of Physicians" by modern medical scholar William Osler. It is as follows: "Inspire me with love for my art and for thy creatures, and in the suffering let me see only the human being."

Golden Ruler

Ronald G. Williams, MD, MPH

L istening to Dr Ronald Williams share his story, our thoughts were drawn to Robert Fulghum and his book, *All I Really Need to Know I Learned in Kindergarten*: "Everything you need to know is in there somewhere. The Golden Rule and love and basic sanitation. Ecology and politics and equality and sane living."[4]

From time to time, just to test the waters to see if his career is on the right track, Ron interviews for a new job. Relating one such recent experience, he elaborates, "About a year ago I interviewed for a medical directorship. The human resource manager who conducted the meeting asked, 'Tell me why you are successful at what you do?' I never thought in those terms before," Ron says. "I told him that he could find a lot of people with credentials similar to mine. What makes me stand out is what my mother taught me about relating to people before I reached the age of 5. She taught us the Golden Rule, to be polite and respectful of other people. Through such basic instruction, we learned to be sensitive to the situations of people." The Golden Rule serves as a foundation for his life.

Before becoming a medical director, Ron practiced pediatrics for about 15 years. Ron served in the US Army for a number of years, practicing initially as a pediatrician. Subsequently, he held a number of positions in research and development and later in operations as an administrator and commander. He is currently the Olympia District Medical Director with Group Health Cooperative in Olympia, Washington.

His participation in this book came from his initial intrigue with our interview request because, if not daily, certainly on a frequent basis, he deals with the issues of soul in medicine. "Initially," he says, "I focused more upon my clinical and technical skills, especially when I was in research and development. However, as I have grown in the position of medical director, the components of soul have become more predominant on almost a daily basis. I am concerned about the interactions between doctors, their patients, and the practice of health care. It's becoming a more important

---

[4] Fulghum R. *All I Really Need to Know I Learned in Kindergarten*. New York, NY: Villard Books; 1989: 7.

component in health care. The dynamics were probably always present, but I didn't appreciate them before this time."

For Ron, the word *soul* represents who he really is at the core of his being. It impacts his leadership style and how he relates to people, guiding his decision-making. "It's a genuine concern for the well-being of others," he reports with enthusiasm. "Kids in particular can see through any false concern for others. Adults can be fooled by it, but like the story of the emperor's clothes, kids seem to know right away if you are genuine. Soul involves empathy tempered with honesty, presenting reality as best we can in a truthful manner. Often it is difficult to wrap empathy and truthfulness in the same package."

Ron sees a connection between soul and spirituality, but not necessarily in a religious sense of the words."Earlier in my life, I would have perhaps said that you could separate these two energies, having one without the other, but I have changed as I have gotten older. Today, I think I would be kidding myself if I believed you could have soul without spirit. They are absolutely linked, because spirituality is an expression of soul. At one point in my life during my high school years, I thought about becoming a minister, but it is probably good that I traveled down another road, because I had difficulty with certain religious concepts. I actually had a local license to preach in the Methodist Church. But like many people, after I went off to college, my religious belief system crumbled. Like Humpty Dumpty, I had to fit the pieces back together again."

According to Ron, there is a close connection between one's body, mind, and spirit, and he believes that the power to heal resides within each individual. As a physician, he brings an expertise, technically and otherwise, to assist the healing process; healing is connected to the totality of a person.

He affirms, "If someone has a disease that causes a physical limitation, we may be able to improve his or her situation through a physical or technological intervention. However, if in a person's mind he or she is unable to accept the limitation, then the healing is only partial. Healing involves the body, mind, and spirit of a person. I can't really separate these elements because they are so linked. You can't deal with just one component to achieve complete healing. Interestingly, I believe a lot of the younger physicians understand what I am speaking about more than some older physicians, who perhaps haven't thought through this issue."

Ron acknowledges that for him personally, the relationship between prayer and healing has been an evolutionary concept. As he says, "It's been one of those revelations that has taken a long time to emerge. I started out as a young man in high school thinking that prayer was everything because I was going to become a minister. Then in college, I became an atheist. I had to rebuild my understanding and belief system. Today, I see prayer as a very powerful force for certain individuals. However, to my knowledge, I have never had a patient ask me to pray for her or him. I know this has happened to other doctors. I have physicians in my organization who find it quite inappropriate to discuss prayer and spirituality with patients, while other doctors are very free and open in this respect. I do know that you cannot force the subject upon a patient if they are not receptive to it. It's an individual matter, each physician bringing or not bringing his or her level of spirituality to the practice."

Like all physicians, Ron is deeply aware of the chaos and turmoil in medicine today. Responding to the comment by some physicians on the trauma in the medical profession, he states, "I think it depends upon how you define being traumatized and to what degree. I don't believe doctors more than other people experience abuse. They are representative of a general population that is traumatized in one form or another. However, MDs as a group do face significant change today."

In his current role, Ron often counsels physicians who face medicine's accelerating change and transition. He laughs, "It seems like that is my job. In many respects counseling with physicians means being a sympathetic listener and making certain that I understand their issues. In many situations, personal issues surface such as family concerns. In other instances, discussions revolve around professional issues, not only in terms of a specific individual concern, but also where we are generally heading in health care. One of the things I do is to assure them that what they are feeling at the moment is a result of the horrendous changes we are facing professionally today. Some doctors say the words and think they understand it, but sometimes they don't dwell deeply enough to get at the root issues. Also, I really want to make sure they understand that this change is occurring nationwide in our profession as well as in other fields. They share these feelings with most of their colleagues. The world is not rose-like in one location or specialty and different in others. Along these lines, we occasionally bring in speakers who have moved toward what they thought were greener pastures, only to find out they weren't very green, just a little different."

Recognizing the growing need for peer support, physician support groups are forming across the country. Although he recognizes this as a vital need today, Ron does not believe enough formal support groups exist for them. "We encourage doctors to engage in smaller group meetings where issues can be discussed. In many cases, it is simply a venting process. In a group practice such as ours, we have the ability to form such groups, but I'm not certain that other physicians have the same luxury. Others may not be feeling the impact of managed care as much, but with us, if a physician becomes too overwhelmed, we have mechanisms of support."

Ron's evolving medical career was rooted in his own childhood experiences. "My father was an administrator in a very small, rural hospital. I grew up around medicine and physicians. I think they had a fundamental imprint upon me in terms of the caring for people and of seeing how people appreciated that care. I went off to college deciding to enter education and become a teacher. But after 2 years, I refocused upon wanting to take care of people medically. I changed my major to pre-medicine and was accepted into medical school. My plans were to return to my hometown of Ottawa, Illinois, as a general practitioner."

He then recalls, "I remember sitting through the second or third day of medical school. One of the professors stood before us and said that all of us who had such plans should drop them, because it simply won't happen. The vast majority of us would specialize and end up somewhere else."

Proving his professor right, Ron did just that. "I specialized in pediatrics because of the influence of some of my mentors. I respected them and during clinical rotations, they made pedi-atrics come alive for me. And, fundamentally, I really liked chil-dren. It was a real fulfillment for me to affect some kind of a cure in them. Various types of people migrate to different specialties. I consider myself to be a people person and those skills especially come into play in pediatrics."

Ron went to medical school at the University of Illinois and completed his residency at Presbyterian St. Luke's Hospital in Chicago. He continues, "I did a rotating internship at a county hospital in Detroit, then came back to Chicago for my pediatric residency. It was during the Vietnam War and I entered the military as a pediatrician, planning to remain for only a few years. However, I remained in the Army for 24 years; that's another story," he laughs. "I had residencies and fellowships in research, but became more and more administrative in my duties. As a reward for my skills in this arena, I was sent to the US Army War College in Carlisle, Pennsylvania. I left there to a command position for a large medical activity."

At that point, Ron says he engaged in some career transitioning. "The question became, did I want to make the final push to become General, or did I want to prepare for life after the military? Fortunately, the Army sent me through another training program. I went to John Hopkins to get a masters in Public Health followed by a year's residency in preventive medicine in Washington State. Two and a half years later I retired from the military."

Ron admits that reconciling his love of people and caring for them as a physician with becoming an administrator is difficult. "Any time you interview a medical administrator, you will find this to be a big struggle in their lives. I still like pediatrics, but think that people skills are very important in administrative medicine. I'm becoming more and more convinced that some of my successes as a manager have been due to my ability to relate and communicate with people in an empathetic manner. Sometimes my strengths become overextended and turn into weaknesses [true for all of us], but my ability to be compassionate toward people has made me a better administrator."

Beyond his career direction, Ron says that he has changed in other ways. "As I gained experience in my medical practice, I became more realistic in terms of my expectations and ability to accept my limitations. Coming out of training, I felt fairly omnipotent. I realized rather quickly that there were a whole lot of things that I could not do. I learned to depend on other people. To a certain degree, this happens to a lot of physicians. In fact, you are probably in deep trouble if you don't come to this conclusion."

"I've certainly made my share of mistakes. Some have been more important than others. Earlier on in my career, I would attempt to justify my actions and protect myself. It made life rather miserable for me. Today, it is still extremely painful for me to make a mistake, although I know that it happens, but I am less self-critical. Mistakes are a part of being human. But still, I struggle with a sense of perfectionism."

Like most of us, Ron experienced some setbacks in his career. Reflecting on the past, he reports, "When I was younger and when my career was on the rise, those setbacks seemed to be about not getting a position that I wanted. Or, I took a turn in the road leading to a dead end. However, my career and life continues to move forward and improve. Setbacks are not the end of my career, but often turn out to be the stepping-stone for something better. You hear so many times that setbacks open new doors."

He shares one such experience. "Probably the most recent setback had to do with changing jobs and bringing a new managerial style into an organization that didn't appreciate how I was operating. I thought I was fundamentally bringing myself to the job, yet people were saying that my actions were inappropriate. That was very difficult and required a significant amount of soul searching," he admits. "But as I worked though this, I realized there was merit to the criticisms. Almost always something good merges from such an experience. Actually, I've probably learned more from my mistakes than from any success I have experienced, as painful as it is."

"I know that for every door that closes, another door opens. But, man! These hallways are a bitch!"

— T-shirt motto

The possibility of leaving his current role and doing something else in his career is not foreign to him. "I think that could happen," he agrees. "I am at a point in my career where I am weighing my options. I am very happy in my current job, but my military duty caused me to move all of the time. I was always given new assignments and tasks. My current job is the longest time I've ever spent in one position and I struggle with my own restlessness. I can see myself performing another job in the medical arena. It would be administrative because I've lost a lot of my pediatric skills, even though I still go to the clinic and see kids. I can evaluate illnesses and conduct physicals, but I've lost touch with the knowledge required in pediatrics today."

"One of the jobs I have looked at was in the pharmaceutical industry," Ron tells us. "It seemed like a very tempting position and would have been administrative. Most of the opportunities for a person like myself are in managed care at the moment. If I would change jobs, it would be something like I am doing now but with a different twist. I never say no when the telephone rings. I gave myself that promise a long time ago. I always look into an opportunity."

Some statistics indicate that fewer young people are considering entering medicine today, and we asked Ron for his perspective. "I've thought a lot about this because of the turmoil in our profession," he responds. "My daughter contemplated medicine, and I encouraged it. I think medicine is a great and noble profession. The joys that come from medicine are difficult to attain in any other profession. I told my daughter that the structure of medicine is uncertain in terms of the future. I suggested that if you are looking at medicine as a means to become rich, you may or may not become well off financially. However, if you are entering the profession because of a sincere desire to care for people, then by all means enter it."

Ron's comments underline his optimism about the future of medicine, although he somewhat qualifies his stance. "I believe there will always be physicians to take care of people. We provide a tremendous service; regardless of the structure or system, it will always be present. Some of the advances that we will be making in the next decade or so will be mind boggling with the breaking of the genetic code and what technology will bring."

"Pessimism is learned helplessness."

— Martin Seligman
Learned Optimism
(1990)

"On the other hand, the profession as it was when I entered it is almost gone. We were sole practitioners back then, with some physicians practicing over the corner drugstore as private entrepreneurs. But, this aspect of medicine is changing, including organization and payment systems. Managed care gets blamed for a lot of things in medicine, but if it didn't exist there would still be a great amount of change. We would probably place blame on another development. And yet," Ron remarks sadly, "managed care often discounts the humanity of doctors as well as their patients. It tends to force medicine into a Detroit-like assembly line. All of the change occurring in medicine these days seems to overpower consideration of the more fundamental issues of soul and spirit in medicine."

Ron maintains, "The core principles of medicine will always exist. Whether our current structure will continue, well, I doubt it. But, we will survive regardless of the structure."

Articles in health care industry publications suggest that California, in particular, is losing physicians at record numbers due to their increasing frustration. We asked Ron to comment on such reports.

"I'm not that familiar with them," he responds. "But, there are two issues driving the situation. There is a decrease in doctors' incomes and a growing sense of losing one's autonomy. I don't see these issues disappearing, not just in California, but also in practically every place where medicine is practiced. We struggle with the issue of autonomy all the time. I get a little frustrated over this concern, because in good [managed care] plans, physicians are making the decisions and not insurance executives. Also, we need to look critically at some of these decisions, because some of them involve waste. It is unethical not to address this problem. For example, there is a significant discrepancy in the C-section rate across the country depending on geographic location. The same thing is true with hysterectomy rates. If you live in certain areas of the US, you may have a 25% or more chance of having a hysterectomy. You can't tell me that has to do with a difference in disease. It involves the way medicine is practiced. Such issues must be addressed. If physicians don't address them, someone else will."

> "Autonomy can be divided into two kinds of freedom—freedom from something and freedom to do something."
>
> — Immanuel Kant
> The Philosophy of Kant (1949)

We asked Ron what advice he would give to a struggling physician who was thinking about leaving the profession. He replies thoughtfully, "Recently I visited with a doctor who has been struggling with the very ideas we have been discussing. He is a fine family practitioner who is concerned not so much about his income but a loss of autonomy. He is struggling with whether he can fit his values and expectations into the current health care environment. Blessed with many interests, he ponders over his options. He finds himself thinking about his life beyond medicine. I worked with him in a supportive manner for a period of time, encouraging him to explore his alternatives. It's much healthier to bring the conflicts to the surface as opposed to hiding them. I also recommended that he not short circuit the process and make any snap decisions."

Ron continues, "The basic issue is exploring what you really want to do with your vocational life. If a doctor takes the time to complete this journey and decides to remain in medicine, then he or she will come back to it with a deepening passion. I remember when I was in the military seeing people leaving the armed services and entering private medical practice. After a number of years they often came back to me wanting to reenlist. They ended up being far more comfortable and receptive to the military environment."

Ron underlines his opinion that many physicians would respond very favorably to a program that offers them an opportunity to explore career alternatives in the midst of the current chaos in medicine. He says, "In our organization, we provide doctors with a sabbatical that can serve to evaluate and renew career direction. Doctors are given a chance to take a leave and do whatever they wish. Sometimes they practice medicine in a Third World country. When they return, they often speak about having a renewal of commitment to medicine. They see the sabbatical as one of the greatest benefits we have to offer them."

"Obviously, doctors in private practice would have a difficult time taking such a leave because their income is tied to seeing patients. Some of them do not even take vacations. They experience unacknowledged burnout, truly a difficult way to live."

ARTISTIC-ORIENTED CAREGIVERS

"[Medical wisdom] is the capacity to comprehend a clinical problem at its mooring, not in an organ, but in a human being."
—Bernard Lown

Connecting With Soul Stories

Emily R. Transue, MD

As we maintain and demonstrate throughout this book, one of the more enduring ways to connect with soul is through stories. Writing about them heightens this connection. Our dialogue with Dr Emily Transue begins with one of her patient-related stories titled "Barcelona."

> I was angry with Mr Stone before I even met him. He had come in to the hospital the day before, with a massive pulmonary embolism. He collapsed at his son's house, was brought in by the medics. A spiral CT of his chest showed a saddle embolism—a huge clot lodged in his pulmonary vein, cutting off blood flow to both his lungs. He was given thrombolytics, powerful clot-dissolving drugs that were developed for treating heart attacks and are experimental in pulmonary embolism. His response was near miraculous; the clot dissolved, his blood pressure and oxygen levels rose, he woke up.
>
> He was moved to the step-down unit, a kind of halfway point between ICU care and the regular ward, and now the ICU team wants to transfer him to my team, the ward team. My resident argues briefly with the ICU resident—he doesn't sound stable, he's still got very abnormal labs and unsteady vitals, shouldn't they watch him for another day? —then gives in and accepts the transfer. All morning, busy with other work, I get called every 15 minutes because his pressure is low or his stats are dropping or his electrolytes are off. I haven't even had time to talk to him yet, much less review his chart. I'm fuming at the unit team for doing this to me, at my resident for accepting it, at the system for allowing, for creating this kind of situation.
>
> But all this melts away the moment I walk into his room. He's a small man, seeming dwarfed by the big hospital bed. He has huge gray-blue eyes, round and gentle, a thoughtful face, and a winning smile. He's extremely thin, and the combination of his slender paleness, his gentle eyes and smile, and his flowing white beard give him a beatific appearance. I feel as if I should kneel and kiss his ring, or perhaps reach out to polish his halo.

The remainder of the story recounts the closeness that develops between the two of them as Mr Stone faces his battle with lung cancer. Emily's words become a journal, capturing her personal feelings as she deals with the ultimate death of this patient. She closes with these words:

> We are talking—he in his now accustomed loud whisper—about his friends in Barcelona, about the dinners they would have, the wonderful food and wine, how they would sit in front of the fire and argue into the night about politics and history.
>
> "I wish I would be able to talk again. . . ." His eyes are filled with an ineffable sadness, wistfulness, and I realize again how suddenly all this came upon him. He felt fine until a month ago; and now he'll never speak aloud again.
>
> "I'm so sorry," I say, squeezing his hand, my eyes filling unexpectedly with tears.
>
> "Bless you," he whispers.
>
> He says, "Bless you" again, the day he goes home, as we are saying good-bye. I want to say, "You have blessed me, more than you know"— But I'm afraid it will sound silly, so I try to put the thought in my eyes instead. I think he understands. He squeezes my hand one last time.
>
> Other patients come, to fill his empty room, to fill my hours. But he stays with me, in the blue sky, in the lush greens and pinks of the spring that has finally come. I remember to look out the windows, to watch the evening light on the cathedral, which I still imagine as being magically transported from Barcelona. And I hold his Spanish islands in my heart when there are moments I have trouble bearing, promising myself that I will go there some-day, that I will walk along the cobbled paths and feel the sunshine and know the joy in my life that he had in his.[1]

At the time of our interview, Emily was preparing to begin her internal medicine career with a fairly large, 80-physician multi-specialty group practice. Listening to her talk, it is hard to believe her limited years of medical experience. It became obvious that her intense desire to connect with others lay at the core of her passion for medicine.

"I love listening to people; it's my biggest joy," she states earnestly. "I love hearing people's stories and getting to know

---

[1] Transue ER. "Barcelona." Used with permission.

them, understanding what they've been through and how they experience things. A huge number of people seem to need to be listened to as part of the process of healing. I think allowing such storytelling to occur is one of the greatest gifts I have to offer."

Emily had no physician role models in her family. "I studied biology as an undergraduate and planned to go to graduate school," she says. "I enjoyed learning about research, but realized I didn't want to be stuck in a lab the rest of my life. I did some research with monkeys and enjoyed working with them." She laughs as she confesses, "I sort of half-jokingly said that people were also primates; it might be interesting to work with them medically as well." And so, she entered medical school.

Emily readily admits that medicine is her passion. She explains, "Like a personal relationship with a family member or friend, medicine can be paradoxically wonderful yet emotionally draining—something you love, but also something not always treating you very well. You seesaw back and forth between excitement and fear of exhaustion. Passion does not always mean bliss or happiness. I love taking care of patients and I love the science of it, but it's very hard, much harder than I thought. There are times when it's hard to maintain the energy level required to do it well. But it's still my passion."

Some experienced physicians refer to the time preceding managed care as the golden age of medicine, lamenting the changing face of health care. As a new physician, Emily perceives it differently. "You hear a lot from long-timers that things aren't like they used to be; today many doctors worry about finances and time pressures. But, I don't remember a time when that wasn't the situation," she says. "I think one of the differences is we younger doctors don't have those memories to look back on."

"Let the counsel of thine own heart stand."

— Ecclesiasticus (190–170 B.L.)

Continuing, she says, "One of my greatest challenges is finding balance and discovering ways to avoid burnout. It's very important to find ways to take of yourself, to get away sometimes, and to dedicate time to do the other things you love in life. And that may be something that younger folks are more aware of, thinking about having families, thinking about whether its necessary to work full time or whether working part time is a viable option."

Emily agrees that lifestyle issues may be more important to people of her generation. "I think I am more conscious of them. Certainly as more women enter medicine, lifestyle surfaces as a significant issue. It's not simply that women are different than men; things are changing for both. The traditional model of the male physician with a wife remaining at home taking care of the kids isn't really working for many people these days. Also, the increase in other pressures pushing doctors to a breaking point forces attention onto lifestyle issues."

Emily's interest in internal medicine evolved during medical school. "I enjoy complicated diagnoses, delving deeply into the cause of things. And, as a primary care physician, you are expected to play a strong and active role in people's health care." Thus, internal medicine seemed to be Emily's best professional specialty.

She confesses, "I never thought about private practice until late in residency. My initial plans revolved around academia, because I really enjoy teaching. My thoughts shifted over time, partly because of knowing a lot of young academic folks who didn't seem very happy. And, I knew I could do a fair amount of teaching in the community, that I could make that a focus without necessarily being in an academic environment."

Emily selected the clinic where she will work based on its operational setting and practice philosophy. She also realized that she wanted to practice in an environment where the connections and relationships between colleagues were highly valued.

She describes the practice environment where she will work as being very traditional. "You have a panel of patients and you are on call for them Sunday through Friday night. If they get sick and go to the hospital, you follow them until they are discharged." She explains, "I am a little frightened about the idea of being tied to a beeper so much of the time. However, this practice setup can be very rewarding. You get to see people through their problems, rather than just handing them off to an on-call or hospital-based person."

Reflecting on her medical journey, Emily admits being naïve about the entire process of becoming a physician. She remarks, "During medical school and residency, I think everybody goes through incredible change." Likening the experience to an accelerated life process, she tries to articulate her feelings. "You experience events most people never see during the course of a lifetime and you face them in a very short number of years. I feel much older today than I did only a few years ago," she reports with some amazement. "It startles me to sometimes run into people who are my age and doing normal late-20s-early-30s things, and to feel very distanced from that. Things that used to seem important just don't anymore." She notes other changes. "I suppose I am a little more jaded than I used to be, a little more self-protective. I used to think that doctors needed to be completely self-sacrificing, that taking care of personal needs was not part of the equation at all. Over time, I realized that that doesn't work. You have to take care of yourself to maintain your ability to care for other people. I value my time much more than I used to. I value having good health. I think a lot more about what it means to have a good life. Everybody has a limited amount of time; you have to use it well."

Emily is both optimistic and pessimistic about medical practice as a whole. "In one sense, I'm very worried. The doctor–patient relationship is an essential piece of medical practice; it's very frightening to watch that being eroded under current time pressures and so on. And, it's scary to realize that it may be possible to become so exhausted that you can't effectively care for people."

"At the same time," she says, "I think most doctors are wonderfully competent and caring people. Many doctors try to protect patients from the pressures of the current health care environment. Ultimately, I predict that things will change when doctors are unable to protect their patients from feeling the effects of those pressures. Then, the pendulum will swing back and the system will have to right itself. The only questions are how long that will take, how bad things will get, and whether, during the low point, I will be able to find a job environment that works for me. But, I think medical care is too important not to get better eventually. Health is something everyone needs. There have always been healers; that won't change."

Emily's blossoming interest in writing springs from her medical experience and training. "When I started my third year of medical school—the first clinical year—I felt myself becoming distanced from the people whom I knew before medicine. It's such a strange life. In a way it's like joining the military and going into battle, having experiences that are foreign to your family and friends. So, like a soldier, I found myself writing a lot of letters to people, to stay connected."

Writing serves another important purpose. Shortly after she began her first clerkship, there was a code and a patient died—the first death of which she'd ever been part. Afterward, she recalls, "I found myself just standing around, not having the faintest idea what to do next, not being able to go on with my day after this incredible thing happened. And yet, no one else seemed to think that it was so significant or unusual." As a way of coping, she wrote about the entire experience and e-mailed it to a friend. Her story received positive feedback from others who read it and was subsequently published.

Writing down her feelings and experiences has been a habit and healing process for Emily, as evidenced in her story, "Barcelona." "I kept writing what I was going through, writing stories about the patients I saw—what I experienced in patient care and what my patients felt." She continued capturing stories throughout medical school and residency. "For me, it's been an essential way of staying connected with my feelings and my thoughts." And, as she says, "It's a way of helping me get these things out of my head; putting them on paper helps me to gain closure. It's also a means to stay connected to people. I have published a few of these stories, and some wonderful responses came from doctors who have been through similar experiences but who hadn't really talked about them." She also found it helpful for patients to learn what their doctor was feeling.

> "[Writing] has given me objectivity and distance so that I can find solid ground, getting my bearing and not being engulfed by the storms which have come again and again in my inner and outer life."
>
> — Morton Kelsey
> Adventure Inward (1980)

Emily's comments remind us of the story of a young man who left his personal journal above a coatrack in a school cafeteria. When he returned to pick it up, it was gone. He fell into despair, petrified at the thought that someone would know and reveal his most intimate secrets. A day or so later, he found the journal returned to the coatrack. On the first page, he read, "Thank you. I didn't know others had thoughts and feelings similar to mine."

As we have noted a number of times, being connected is central to Emily's passion and tantamount to her understanding of the process of healing. While she is uncertain about how to define healing, she believes it to be a bedrock word; you know it when you experience it.

"It means various things at different times," she explains. "People need healing in different ways according to their situations. When they feel better, whether their symptoms go away or not, they are more able to cope. I think the biggest power to heal comes from being interconnected."

While Emily does not pray, she concedes, "People get strength in different ways. I'm sure that prayer is an essential for some people, though not for me." She also believes that spirit can mean different things. She says, "If you think of spirit as being the essential part of you that reaches out to someone else and connects with them, then that is incredibly important. And you have to nurture that part of yourself in whatever way you can. You definitely need to be in a good place yourself to be able to reach out to and help others."

Ultimately, Emily hopes that she will be remembered for making a difference. "I would like to be remembered as someone who helped people take something destructive and turn it into a positive, growth experience. It's amazing to watch how people respond to what happens to them. The same event can be totally devastating or completely transforming for different people. I think that we have the power to help effect the positive outcome, and what I would like to devote my life to doing."

Medicine as Art

James N. Easter, MD

Growing up in a small Indiana town in the 1950s, Dr Jim Easter was not convinced about medicine as a career. As he remembers, several factors ultimately contributed to his decision. "Obviously, it's a good income, though I didn't anticipate getting rich," Jim says. "Being a physician also gains some respect in the community and contributes to a nice social life. But more than that," he explains, "I liked the idea of helping people. My family doctors were the Farrars [two physician brothers] and they talked to me about medicine." Grinning, he adds, "My mother wanted me to have a professional career, though not necessarily to be a doctor. I think she wanted me to be a lawyer. It wasn't until my second or third year in pre-med that I decided I really did want to go into medicine."

Jim spent 35 years in private practice as a family medicine physician until health concerns forced his early retirement. He admits that medicine was originally not a passion in the way he defines the word. "I view passion as an intense emotional feeling drawing you toward an activity. However, once I began practicing medicine, it became a passion." In the days before specialization, Jim loved the broad spectrum of medical care that a general practice afforded. "I especially loved delivering babies," he says enthusiastically. "Nothing in my practice really bored me. The closest thing to being bored was office practice, which is rather silly for a practitioner to admit."

"When I began practicing, I administered anesthesia because I had residency training in that area. I helped in surgery, did OB, and worked in the ER. So, I had a lot of hospital work." He remarks somewhat wistfully, "But as the years went by, specialists took over, and then it became mostly an office practice caring for only a few patients in the hospital. At times, I did get somewhat bored with seeing colds and minor injuries, but not to the point where I considered quitting medicine."

Listening to Jim describe his medical career, it became clear about the importance he placed on the patient–physician relationship. "How you deal with your patients is an art form," he says firmly. "Of course, it isn't true of all young doctors today, but it seems so many young physicians want to rush in, make a diagnosis, and rush out. It may be true of the older ones as well, but more of the younger doctors don't seem to pay enough attention to the other needs of their patients, such as emotional issues."

Jim believes being a good doctor involves more than understanding disease. "Any physician can be trained as a diagnostician," he suggests. "I believe that my best gift was spending time with patients." Admittedly, the longer amount of time he spent routinely with his patients was not viewed by all of his patients in the same positive light. "Because I spent time with my patients, I was slow and methodical as opposed to those physicians who pushed patients out the treatment room. So, those patients who were more interested in getting in and out quickly went to other doctors."

"Medicine may be largely a body of knowledge, but healing is a personal skill."

— Roy Porter
Medicine, A History of Healing
(1997)

Living and working in a small community, Jim acknowledges it was much easier to know his patients' stories. "In a big city, people get lost in the shuffle. A lot of my patients were friends of mine whom I saw socially. Before the community attracted pediatricians, I took care of several of the other doctors' children."

Jim clearly remembers how the importance of taking time with a patient was brought home through a near disaster during his residency. The incident remains fresh in his mind. "I had 3 months of anesthesia training at the medical center before I began practicing. During the last month, I was on call one night, responsible for administering anesthesia in the whole medical center. A child entered and I had to determine the dosage required to tranquilize him for a cardiac catheterization. Because I had other things to do, I was in a hurry and left him after prescribing the dosage. When I came back, the chief resident was really upset. Apparently, this child received a big overdose causing the staff to intubate him. Fortunately the boy did not die, but it was quite a close call. Apparently, I made a mistake in the calculation by misplacing the decimal point and the child got 10 times the correct dosage. It was an honest mistake but it devastated me for quite a while. I even thought, 'Do I want to do this?' Doctors must realize they can make mistakes and mistakes can be disastrous. A good physician doesn't make very many of them or very often."

During the course of his long practice, Jim believes himself fortunate in not facing many setbacks. An initial financial setback occurred when he went from a group to a solo practice. "When I graduated," he explains, "I started in a group of three doctors. Perhaps all of us felt insecure about going out on our own, so we banded together," he smiles. "But, it didn't work out and we finally split up, still maintaining our relationship in that we signed out to each other for coverage. I was on my own, but that really didn't bother me. I liked being an independent physician."

"In terms of other setbacks, I don't think I had any other real ones other than my health. When I was 45, I had a coronary followed by a series of continuing health problems." Emotionally, making the decision to modify his practice was not easy. "The coronary changed my practice. I stopped OB, quit assisting in surgery, and I really stopped everything but hospital and office practice. I ended my hospital practice a few years before I retired."

Acknowledging the changing face of health care, Jim admits to being fairly pessimistic about medicine. "On the one hand," he states, "I am hopeful about medicine as a science and as an art. Although a lot of the younger physicians seem to have lost some of the art of medicine, they certainly are well trained. Technically, I believe the outlook for medicine itself is excellent. We are making great strides every day."

"However," he adds, "as far as the finances and the nonclinical aspects of medicine, I see the outlook as rather bleak." Reflecting on his own practice, he confesses, "I had so many HMOs and PPOs I had to hire extra help. Because of all the employees I needed, my office expense ratio rose from 31% during the first few years of practice to 62% when I left. It was a hassle. I finally retired, not only because of my health, but also because of burnout. But it wasn't a burnout from medicine," he hastens to add. "It was burnout due to the way I had to practice and the governmental restrictions."

"I probably would not recommend medicine to a young person today," he admits reluctantly. "Of course, it would depend on what other fields the young person wanted to consider. Also, I would give them the facts about medicine as I saw it and let them make their own decision. I wouldn't tell them *not* to go into medicine, but I certainly wouldn't encourage them to any great degree. I enjoyed medicine so much for so many years, but then stopped enjoying it. When I closed my office, it had become a drudgery."

If Jim could begin his career again, he believes he would select another path. "I would be a physicist, probably in some kind of research. I loved math and physics, which were more enjoyable than biology. During my undergraduate work, I liked anatomy but not biology. Today, law might be a better profession because it has fewer controls. I probably would have been a good lawyer," he grins, "because I did well in history, government, and speech. However, that wasn't my love."

An excellent, long-time contract bridge player, Jim plays frequently, having recently moved from Indiana to Florida. Although he enjoys the freedom of retirement, with his health stabilized, he finds himself thinking about new vocational options. While state medical licensure and malpractice requirements probably preclude working within health care at any level, Jim's skills and interests can take him in any number of directions.

Jim finds himself in a situation similar to many older physicians (and the older public in general). After a period of time in retirement, boredom might surface. You can only play so many games of bridge or holes of golf each week. With increasing life spans, today the gerontologists are suggesting that, for all practical purposes, senior citizenship begins at age 75, not age 65. So, how do you maintain purpose and passion in life and work as you age?

"To be old is a glorious thing when one has not unlearned how to begin."

— Martin Buber
I and Thou (1970)

In her book, *Don't Stop the Career Clock*, Dr Helen Harkness differentiates between chronological age and functional age.[2] Up until recent times, many people assumed that they must stop functioning vocationally when they reached their mid-60s. However, because of scientific breakthroughs, health care, and improved nutrition, we might expect that, at least careerwise, midlife begins around 60. Because of savings, Social Security, and Medicare, many people find themselves in a position to transition from having a job to having the freedom to follow their vocational passion.

Dr Harkness raises the interesting question, "Knowing what you know about yourself and your world, what would you do with your life and in your work if you could deduct 20 years from your chronological life?" What would you do?

[2] Harkness H. *Don't Stop the Career Clock*. Palo Alto, CA: Davies-Black Publishing; 1997.

When Social Security was formulated in the 1930s and 65 was established as the beginning age to receive benefits, the average life expectancy was around 45. This was during the depression when the unemployment rate was about 25%. Today, retiring at the age of 65 can be a mindless assumption.

For assistance in reinventing your purpose and passion in life, numerous resources are available in terms of career assessment and development. A good place to begin is with Richard Bolles' perennial bestseller, *What Color Is Your Parachute?*[3] In the Appendix, it includes how to find your mission in life. The Internet also offers an abundance of resources.

---

[3] Bolles R. *What Color Is Your Parachute?* Berkeley, CA: Ten Speed Press; 2001.

Creative and Passionate Pathologist

Harry Chinchinian, MD

What immediately strikes us about Harry Chinchinian is his obvious passion for knowledge and his appetite for life-long learning. A successful author of adult mysteries and children's books, Harry signs his children's stories with an artistic characterization of himself as a fuzzy, loveable bear's head. It fits him well.

Currently in his 70s and semiretired from his rural area pathology practice, he still remains somewhat active in the profession, traveling around the area as a locum tenens and teaching. An associate professor of pathology at the College of Pharmacy, Washington State University, he teaches a three-credit course. "You know, " he chuckles, "the best thing about the pathophysiology course is that it's mandatory; they have to take it! That's the best thing—they're pushed into me."

Harry did not intend to be a pathologist. An usual circumstance led to medicine. He began our interview and his journey back through time by pulling out of a bag a black and white photograph of a physician leaning against a counter, drinking coffee, and smoking a cigarette. Harry talks about this particular hero. "When I was in college in 1947, I came across a picture and article in *Life* magazine about Dr E. Guy Ceriani in Kremmling, Colorado, and I was quite taken by them. I was 21. I was in WWII and it was through the GI bill that I got into college. I saw those pictures and knew he had to be a great guy."

Harry contacted Dr Ceriani and subsequently lived with him for a week at the hospital where he worked. "I made rounds with him," Harry recalls. "I helped in surgery. It was extraordinarily kind of him to take me. At that time I was a ski bum in Winter Park, Colorado." After college, Harry met another mentor, Dr George Hoydt Whipple, who was the dean of the medical school at Rochester (NY) and had won a Nobel Prize for his work with pernicious anemia. Pulling out another photo, Harry says, "I became a pathologist because of him. He was immensely kind to struggling students."

Although Harry doesn't believe his passion is pathology, he does agree that he has a passion for medicine. He believes that being a pathologist suits his personality. He is convinced that different medical specialists have their own personality. "We all have a different personality," he states. "Pathologists in general are the types of people who are scholarly," he laughs, quickly adding, "although I wouldn't describe myself as being scholarly."

Once he made the decision to enter pathology, Harry never strayed from that interest because it allowed him to use multiple skills. "Pathology covered everything. You got to do everything. I liked the teaching part; I liked the doing part. I liked knowing, as do most pathologists. I liked knowing exactly what was going on. Pathologists actually get to see the tissue; they actually get to see the cancer and then make the diagnosis. I liked that part. Then there's teaching. You get to teach the nurses and you teach students. So that makes you keep up. You're forced to keep up so they don't ask you questions you can't answer." He laughs, "You try to stay ahead of them by reading everything you can, surgery journals, internal medicine journals, OB/GYN journals. It's fascinating; so you never get bored. It's very rewarding that way."

Harry denies that pathology is his passion because he enjoys everything about medicine as a whole. Instead, he describes his passion as medicine and being helpful. He has a little difficulty defining passion. Somewhat hesitantly, he confesses, "It's an embarrassing word." He sees it as being all-exclusive rather than inclusive and explains, "You can have a passion for many things. I enjoy and have a passion for drawing, painting, sculpture, writing, and music. So all these are my passions as well. Which one is more rewarding than the next? One is self-indulgent and the other may be helpful toward others. So, each passion is different."

Although as a pathologist, Harry's relationship with patients differs from that of other specialties, he believes the qualities of being a good physician are similar.

"I think," he says considering the question, "one quality is craftsmanship; and it's almost true of any field. It's sticking to something, doing a good job of it; coming in everyday, putting in your time from morning to night, and knowing you have to do it. A lot of it may be humdrum and may be routine, although it is possible to do things differently so that 'putting in your time' is no longer routine, fooling yourself so that it isn't routine." Harry punctuates the importance of being present with the example of the outstanding baseball player, Carl Ripkin, Jr, who, in 18 years, played the most consecutive games in baseball history.

Another distinguishing quality Harry believes is doing one's homework. "Doing your homework is more important than anything else." In his role as a pathologist, Harry has frequently been called on to testify in court.

"The good lawyers did their homework," he says. "The poor lawyers never asked me what my findings were and so, to their great surprise, they had to adjourn and go into recess because I surprised them when my findings were completely opposite to what they had expected. They simply hadn't asked." He shakes his head. "You have no idea how many lawyers do that; they simply do not do their homework. I know that is startling. It was startling to me the first time it happened." He chuckles. "We're talking about gunshot wounds, where the bullet entered and exited, that type of thing, or what the blood alcohol level was or wasn't. You have to do your homework."

Perhaps surprisingly to others, on a daily basis, Harry finds wonder and mystery in pathology. "Everyday is different because the tissues you receive from surgery are from different people. So every tissue you get is different, although the diagnosis may be similar in many cases." He elaborates. "Because each cancer acts differently, you have to grade each cancer differently. For example, you have to keep thinking whether this is going to metastasize or not, or whether this is simply benign and a simple incision will take it out. These are the decisions that the pathologist makes for the surgeon."

Although as a practicing pathologist Harry rarely has direct patient contact, he is still an integral part of a patient's care team. He takes phone calls from physicians continuously asking for advice about patients who have a particular rash or a lump or how to interpret a lab result.

"We get about 40 calls a day," he says. "I don't have patients, but yet in a sense I do. I am visualizing this patient because the physician is describing this patient. 'This patient is short, fat, thin, eats excessive amounts. This patient looks like a hyperthyroid. This patient had cancer 3 years ago, and now there is a lump here, what do you think?'"

Although Harry finds it difficult to separate soul from a religious context, he has less difficulty in talking about the power to heal and the role of spirit and prayer in healing. He believes that the power to heal resides in an individual's own immune system controlled in many ways by the mind. He sees spirit and prayer playing a "great role" in the healing process.

"That's what I meant when I talk about the mind being the controlling factor. The optimists, the people who want to get better, even insist on getting better, heal quicker. For those who are pessimistic or depressed, the immune system doesn't kick in to heal them."

Harry is definitely hopeful about the future of medicine. "It's going to change," he states emphatically. "Everybody's role in it is going to change. Right now we have fractionated the patient into pieces so that if you have this, you get this specialist and he only looks at that part. It's a false fractionation. But," he concedes, "it's difficult to be an expert in all fields. I think there's going to be more and more overlap as time goes on and less ultraspecialization."

Acknowledging the general chaos in medicine today and the pessimism of some physicians leaving the field, Harry adds, "Perhaps they've lost sight of their original goal and that was to take care of patients." He is concerned about HMOs and what he terms political maneuvering to get free prescriptions and free physician care.

"There's no free lunch," he cautions. "Somebody has to spend the time and put in the work to learn to do the things a physician does." He fears that in an effort to short cut the process, paying less money for fully qualified medical professionals, patient care will ultimately be compromised.

Having talked at length about his passion for medicine, it is time to look at another side of this talented physician. Referring to some of the earlier passions he identified, his eyes twinkle, and he laughs generously at himself, admitting to feeling a little embarrassed about references to his talents and gifts. "I call them nutty obsessions, not really passions. I have a very tolerant wife who allows me to do all these things instead of doing important things."

Harry does not see himself as having exceptional gifts and talents for writing, art, music, and gardening. "I just enjoy what I do," he says demurring the compliment. "That's not fair," he says, " because I am enjoying myself. I'm having fun. I have a great wife, wonderful kids, everything. I have been very lucky. Pure luck."

Harry began writing as a child. He recalls, "I have always written as far back as I remember. As a little child I was writing. I was drawing pictures with crayons. Nobody understood what I was drawing," he smiles. "I was drawing, I was convincing them it was what I said it was."

Harry has written a series of adult mysteries and a short selection of children's books that he also illustrated. The mysteries, Harry tells us, feature a forensic pathologist and are for the general public. "That's not difficult because that's my job with forensics. We did all the autopsies for the coroner. There is one mystery after another of why and how a person dies. That's easy to do. Writing children's stories is much more of a challenge and tickles me. It is an embarrassment to write mystery stories when there are so many wonderful mystery writers out there that I couldn't hold a candle to. I admire several mystery writers that do a wonderful job."

His children's books grew out of a love for his grandchildren. "I never stopped writing things for the grandkids. I try to write the stories for a particular child using their expressions and their idioms and the way they look at life. What worked with Nick would not work with Holly or with her sister. Her sister is a straight A student and likes formal things and precision. Holly is a 'punch them out if they get in your way.' I had fun with all these stories, fitting them to their different personalities."

The stories were only published because of Harry's recovery from coronary bypass surgery almost 10 years ago. "Right after the surgery, I couldn't do anything. I couldn't think. I could hardly get out of bed to walk 3 feet. I was getting depressed that I wasn't able to do anything. My daughter said, 'Why don't you publish those stories?'" He agreed because it would give him something to think about that required no real effort since they were already written.

He continues to write stories for the boys now that the girls are older. Though he plans to continue writing adult mysteries, he does not plan to publish additional children's books. "They are really for that particular child. I don't think they have enough general interest for others," he says.

Harry does not paint to show, only for enjoyment. Both art and his music are, as he puts it, "to amuse myself." Believing he plays badly, he chuckles, "I've been at the piano, guitar, banjo, squeeze-box. Anything that makes a sound that will drive you crazy, I will pick it up and start playing."

In his art, Harry explains his preferences. "My preference is pen and ink. I like color. I also like pencil drawings. I enjoy what you can do. It fascinates me that you can take an ordinary pencil and by using it lightly, or darkly, you can create three-dimensional things. I get a kick out of watercolor because it is quick, it's easy, and it's best to know what you are going to do before you do it. Oil is my favorite because you can put so many nuances in oil, so many colors."

Harry and his daughter just returned from an oil painting workshop taught by a well-known colorist. Laughingly, he tells about the class. Describing the artist, he says, "His colors are so stunning. I don't know any other person who has the colors that he does in his oil paintings. He was helping me with my painting and said, 'Think like a child.' I told him, all my life I've had to be meticulous and careful, and now you are telling me to throw paint on and be daring and be a child!"

Listening to Harry's story, we are struck by a common thread of creativity that runs through everything he does. Whether it is writing a story, drawing a picture, playing music, planting a garden, or finding the right answers from the information at hand as a pathologist, elements of creativity are present in each.

Admitting that there are so many things in which he delights, Harry says, "In fact, I delight so much in certain favorite writers that I read one chapter of their book a day so as to prolong it. That's what I did with the Harry Potter series; I only read one chapter a day. I didn't want it to end."

Harry immensely enjoys whatever he is doing at that particular moment in time. Whether it is aerobics, painting, pulling weeds in his garden, or writing, he fully engages himself.

"That's true in life," he says. "Life is so short. You need to enjoy it. You have to have that sort of philosophy in life; enjoy things."

PHYSICIANS WITHOUT SHINGLES

Spouse Perspectives

Physicians Without Shingles

Physician Spouse Perspectives

Because of their often intimate involvement in health care, we thought it only appropriate to include a few brief interviews with physicians' spouses, especially those associated with the American Medical Association Alliance. As a volunteer arm of the AMA, comprised of physicians' spouses, the Alliance is dedicated to promoting better health, ensuring sound health care legislation, and fund-raising for medical education.

At least in some ways, many spouses are physicians without shingles. Sharon Seaman, whose husband Richard is an otorhino-laryngologist (ear, nose, throat) in Olympia, Washington, laughingly asserts, "So many times we serve on the front line. People approach us in the grocery stores and at the soccer games wanting to know who to go to for a particular problem or need. They report to us about a child being sick for 3 weeks or so, and we tell them that we are not physicians, but are able to make suggestions as to which doctor they might see. I suppose people assume that we have almost the same knowledge as our spouses."

Written by Emily Hill during her term as president of the Florida Medical Association Alliance, the following article bears witness to the reality that physician spouses are often intimately aware of today's pressures on physicians:

Requiem

A good doctor died today. He treated each patient with kindness and respect, listened with real interest to their tales of "which fish got away" and "how big the rack was on that buck;" mourned their losses, celebrated their victories. He went to the office early, came home far too late, and repeated it all again the next day. He worked the ill into an already overbooked schedule and never asked if a patient could pay. ("The poor get sick, too," he would say.) His nurses adored him—quite possibly because he respected them—as did the hospital staff, since he never asked anyone to do anything he would not do himself. He volunteered for hospital positions, volunteered in the community, and did it all with the idea that this was his way of giving thanks for the gift he had been given to practice medicine. The doctor was happy and so was the doctor's family; for even though they missed him, they were proud of his ethics as well as his accomplishments. But then, things began to change. The doctor's ability to treat his patients was slowly eroded by insurance companies and accountants who looked at bottom lines rather than outcomes; and the ever-present threat of lawsuits turned patients from friends to potential litigants. His clinics swelled to unmanageable proportions. Since the clinic where he practiced took more, the doctor had to see more and more patients just to keep his head above water. He saw things that needed to be changed in his practice, but he was removed from committees when he brought the issues to light. A deep sadness soon settled over the doctor; his family saw it; his friends saw it; the doctor just kept denying it. "Patients have to be seen; no one else will see them," he would say. "Who will see them if I don't?" The peace that he once found practicing medicine was replaced by a sullen anger that ate away at his soul. He tried desperately to control his situation, but the events of his life were beyond control. His friends—the few who remained—tried to reach him; his family, frantic about his health, begged him to retire. But the doctor just kept plugging away, always believing that if he worked just a little harder, did things just a little better, his life would turn around and everything would be okay. And then it happened . . . one morning the doctor just didn't wake up. The medical examiner said it was heart failure, but his family knew better . . . the doctor had succumbed to a 'death of the spirit' long before and the physical passage was just a secondary result. He was killed by a system he neither understood nor had the tools to manage. He died because he tried to play a game whose rules did not mesh with his own abilities or code of ethics. He died of a broken heart.[1]

Emily states, "This story reflects a composite of people and, more than that, a composite of emotions. We in organized medicine take time from our schedules, commit hours we don't have, and spend funds for which we will never be reimbursed to fight battles for medicine. We do this for all the good doctors present and future that deserve a life that celebrates, not denigrates, their sacrifices as well as their accomplishments. And we remember this good doctor who gave so much and deserved so much better."

Emily's husband was forced by financial and practice circumstances to leave his practice in Pensacola after 19 years. On his last day in the office, Emily relates, he literally wept, not for himself, but for his patients. She affirms, "This is why I love him and why, after 29 years of marriage, he is still my hero." They subsequently moved to South Carolina to continue practicing medicine.

---

[1] Emily Hill, Past President Florida Medical Association Alliance, reprinted with permission.

Sharon views Emily's article as descriptive of some of the changes she has seen in her husband. She knows about the added stress firsthand because she volunteers in the office, handling accounts payable. In his 60s and beginning to slow down, Richard no longer performs surgery, but sees patients in his office. "Currently, it works out well because he loves interacting with patients," she reports. An office manager will eventually replace Sharon, but she will continue to volunteer her services in the local community and beyond.

As a generalization, Sharon doesn't necessarily agree that most physicians' spirits are diminishing because of the chaos in health care. However, she acknowledges that many spouses spend numerous hours fighting battles for medicine. With a voice filled with concern, she states, "We do it for those who are doctors today and for the future practitioners. I am concerned about having adequate care for my grandchildren and for those of us entering our senior years."

Sharon says, "At least in the past, one of the beauties of having an organized AMA Alliance is they truly reach out and welcome new medical families. It provides an incredible network to meet people and enter a support system. Also, we commit ourselves to the greater community improving health care and education."

Continuing, she relays, "In 1982, I became the county chapter president. It allowed me to participate in a wonderful training program conducted by the national AMA Alliance staff in Chicago. It was an intensive course in meeting management and on how to become involved in legislative affairs. I made friends with people throughout the United States, relationships that continue to this day. I was also introduced to a variety of health projects such as supporting the use of seat belts and infant seats. We also promoted such initiatives as smoke-free hospitals and wearing of medical alert identification in case of a medical incident happening to you while out in public."

Today, a major Alliance issue revolves around violence. Sharon asserts, "About 4 years ago we began a SAVE program, meaning 'Stop America's Violence Everywhere.' It operates as a joint project between the AMA and the Alliance. During 1 week in October, we promote activities throughout the country, often related to 'shelter showers' where we gather items to be donated to local shelters for woman and children. Often such people leave their homes with nothing but the clothes they are wearing. We also do things like publishing coloring books for children that focus upon self-esteem and the prevention of violence between children. Our national organization provides a wealth of resources to call upon."

Unfortunately, at the beginning of 2001, the Washington State Alliance closed its doors. About 5 to 10 years before this, a new generation of physician families moved into communities with dual careers. Also, female spouses began refusing affiliation with an organization perceived to be supportive of and subservient to their husband's profession; women wanted their own identity.

Sadly, Sharon asks, "How can you remove yourself from some of the pain your mate currently experiences in health care practice? He or she often brings it home every evening. If it is not impacting you financially, it must impact you emotionally. But we experienced a generation who refused participation and, consequently, we lost the potential pool of county leaders interested in moving to the state level. When I was state president 10 years ago, we had 19 county chapters totaling 1,200 active members; today that figure drops to 4 counties with about 400 people. So we removed the state link between the counties and the national office."

Apart from having dual careers, Sharon notes another factor affecting participation in the Alliance, namely the current competition and divisiveness among providers. "Earlier, people cooperated and worked together on projects because the task at hand was the main focus," she affirms. "However, today physicians may be at odds with one another. Doctors compete with one another in the clinical arena and this impacts how their spouses relate personally to one another. This causes us to center our attention on rebuilding the foundation of friendships and support, especially during these current times of change and chaos. With acquisitions, mergers, clinic closures, and the ever-present possibility of malpractice suits, this foundation of collegiality and mutual backing is more vital than ever before."

Sharon spoke about how physicians often bring a lot of anger and frustration home in the evening. There needs to be time spent together speaking about daily work experiences. "I can't see a marriage surviving without such sharing," she emphasizes. "Some physicians such as neurosurgeons and oncologists deal with unpleasant outcomes, and these have to weigh upon them. You can't escape the grief."

Over the course of our writing, we received a number of e-mails from physicians' spouses who responded to how the incidents of loss and grief impact their relationships. Some people asked not to be identified by name. One such individual wrote, "My husband and I share our day's events with one another. Initially, I was unaware of the impact it had on him when he would tell me he had diagnosed another patient with cancer. However, after listening to him over time, I have grown to realize how this makes him feel helpless at times. Being there for him to express his feelings and helping him through these times has only brought us closer, but helps him to accept certain outcomes and deal with the grief process. Listening has become a *very* important part of being the spouse of a physician. Their lives are filled with life-and-death situations; most of our family problems or situations are not life and death. Prioritizing reality, feelings, and emotions is very important when dealing with our own family situations."

Another spouse reports, "I feel the experience of loss and grief impacts each physician differently, depending on personality, outlook on life, and how emotional issues were handled during childhood. I have had great difficulty being the person who receives the brunt of the 'saved' emotions. Attempting to share a life with someone who lives in denial and who has a perfectionist orientation is quite challenging."

It helps for the spouse to actually work in the practice office, if only part-time, Sharon believes. She reports, "No one knew that I was the doctor's wife, so I got to relate to some of the more irate patients who couldn't understand why they had to wait for an appointment or why we couldn't see them because they had no referral or health insurance card. Also, when the charts begin to stack up, the tension builds in the back hall and little irritations begin to build."

"In any case, it's never boring. Actually, it's really fun because every day is different. Also, Richard and I worked with one another in such areas as the medical political arena, traveling together to meetings. I look forward to that because it becomes very stimulating to gather with other people."

One of Sharon's skills is forming coalitions, bringing people together for important causes. As a field director for the AMA Alliance, she was responsible for activities in six states. She especially enjoys connecting with others as they address common issues. Aware of it or not, we suspect she enhances soul among people, because soul is all about such connections.

"Soul is that which makes me alive, my reason for being," she underlines. "And, in addition to being a soul-oriented person, I'm also an angel fan. I firmly believe we all have a guardian angel, constantly working with us as a kind of copilot."

Sharon and Richard continue to share quality time together. They golf, spend time together with the grandchildren, and, until recently, sailed together. With three boys, sailing especially had been a big part of their lives.

We asked Sharon to share her views regarding the future of health care. She responded, "I guess because I'm an optimist, my hope is that we will return to the earlier, wonderful days of physician–patient relationships. I hope the doctors can get back to practicing medicine, allowing the business aspect of it to be taken care of by someone else. Through the Alliance, we attempt to influence our legislators and to elect people who are friends of medicine."

Barbara Ellman also works to influence legislators. She reports, "I am the wife of a physician who practiced OB-GYN for almost 30 years and has been in a new partnership for the past 2 years doing GYN oncology. It has been quite a shift, from what is basically a happy field of medicine with good outcomes, to a field that frequently produces terminally ill patients with poor prognosis. We have been married 19 years, the first 16 of which I worked in my husband's office as the practice/business office manager. When my husband made the decision to become very involved in medical-legal issues and to become an active lobbyist/advocate for medicine and for his patients, I decided that if I did not become involved as well, our marriage would suffer. For the past 15 years, we have worked hand in hand, fighting for the medical system that we believe is best for patients and for physicians. We volunteered our time as lobbyists for the Medical Society of the State of New York and built relationships with our legislators and government officials. I now work full-time for the medical society as a lobbyist, and my husband still devotes his days off and vacation time to efforts involving patient and physician advocacy. We like to think that we have made a real impact on legislation that has passed or been defeated in our state. It is a passion that we share, and has helped strengthen our relationship over the years."

Barbara affirms, "My husband is a very 'hands on' physician and has frequently gone with his patients when they have had

biopsies or other procedures. If they are facing difficult surgery
by another physician and need someone to hold their hand, he
has gone to the operating room with them and stayed with them
until they have been anesthetized. His patients love him, and it is
not uncommon for them to call our home at any time if they need
his support or advice."

"It is a difficult and thankless profession in many ways,"
Barbara reports. "However, I understand how important it is for
someone as caring as he is to do exactly what he does. I saw my
husband spend an entire evening in our home with the father of a
31-year-old woman with breast cancer, helping him to understand
the disease and to know what to expect. He assisted in getting the
best surgeons, oncologists, etc, to take care of her. Or, I hear him
on the phone night after night giving support to a 40-year-old
woman with breast cancer who is undergoing chemotherapy."

At times, Barbara wishes her husband had chosen a different
career. "However," reflecting upon it she states, "that would
deprive his many patients of exactly the kind of physician we
would all want to have for ourselves. It would also deprive him
of the satisfaction he must get from knowing that he has made
such a difference in people's lives, medically, emotionally,
and psychologically."

Not all physician spouses are so blessed. A past president of a
state Medical Society Alliance group shares, "My husband and I
were on our honeymoon when he received his acceptance to
medical school; therefore, I have been with him from the start.
He finally went into practice as a radiologist the week of our
tenth anniversary. There were 4 years of med school, a 1-year
general rotating internship (that sounds antique!), 2 years in the
Air Force during Vietnam (he was stationed at Lowry Air Force
Base in Denver), and a 3-year radiology residency. He was board
certified when he finished, and a year later was board certified
in ultrasound. Those certifications required three board exams,
one each year for 3 years. They were a tremendous strain on
all of us."

She continues, "One night shortly after the last board exam
I was coming down the stairs after putting the children to bed.
Partway down the stairs I stopped, alert that something was
wrong in the house. I paused, assessing what was not in order.
It took a few moments to realize that the house was simply quiet.
It jolted me to realize we had lived so long with the voice on the

tape recorder detailing the sample X rays that my husband studied night after night. It was no longer part of our lives."

"A year earlier I had told him that he had engaged in tunnel
vision for 10 years. His eyes became so focused on his goal to be a
board-certified physician that the children and I were outside his
range of vision. I, like many other physicians' wives, felt and
often acted like a single parent. For so many years he was
unavailable and never really became part of the family."

"We are now grandparents. As much as I would like to think
that he will become involved with the grandchildren, he still
remains distant in great part because he continues to work full-
time (we're only 56) and his schedule grows in severity as time
goes on. . . . We live well, but it has come with a high price." In a
later e-mail, she informed us that they entered therapy and now
the situation has improved.

This woman's testimony provides a sad but timely bridge into
our section on strategies for taking care of oneself, where we will
provide strategies for healing past wounds and for reclaiming
soul in life, its many relationships, and in health care.

CONCLUDING REFLECTIONS

Jim's Concluding Reflections

I wish this book had been published 6 months or so before my 94-year-old father passed away in June of 2000. I know he would have read it. It would have made for interesting and, perhaps healing, discussions.

For example, as Bob Barnes suggests, a good physician is not only technically competent, but also naked, stripped of wearing a mask of power and perfection. My father liked his family physician of 10 years, and we both knew he was medically competent. During the last few weeks of his life we visited him together because of Dad's great pain from a bleeding bladder that was impacted by his prostate cancer. Doc Smith (not his real name) certainly talked a lot. In fact, he was one of the fastest speakers I've ever heard. Too bad. Along with many others, Dub Howard suggests that a good doctor first listens to a patient, "a rare bird these days." Perhaps Doc Smith was feeling pressure because of managed care, although Dad was not enrolled in an HMO. In any case, I felt rushed, especially when we all knew this could be the beginning of the end of his life. In retrospect, instead of him, I wish almost any of the doctors interviewed for this book could have cared for him.

My father was in so much pain he could hardly sit down, yet Doc Smith didn't want to give him any medication because he said it would blunt the mind. Finally, he relented and shortly thereafter we had great hamburgers and conversation at his favorite restaurant. It was our last meal together.

Lon Hatfield states, "Sometimes the ultimate healing for a person is in death." Not long after we ate those hamburgers, Dad's kidneys stopped functioning and he went to ICU. After an initial examination, the consulting nephrologist recommended a kidney biopsy. No one explained that it represented one of two options, the second one being to let nature take its course as per the instructions in his living will. However, we never explored this option. He could have remained on dialysis for a few weeks, gone back to the retirement home, and said good-byes to his family and many friends. We could have enlisted hospice care for 4 weeks instead of 4 days. However, he decided to proceed with the invasive surgery.

Upon returning from the surgery, communication ceased for all practical purposes. Occasionally, Dad was aware of my sister's and my presence, but he spoke hardly a word. It was also obvious that he was very uncomfortable. The staff had to tie his hands to the sidebars to keep him from pulling out the tubes. After a week, the kidney biopsy report came back negative, meaning no damage was detected. The nephrologist recommended keeping him on dialysis for a month or more, hoping that the kidneys would function again. I guess he was trained to keep people alive at all cost. However, after great struggle over the options, my sister and I decided, as they say, to "pull the plug." Thereafter, the only comment the nephrologist offered was to say that he was taking himself off the case. Later, Doc Smith phoned to affirm our decision and said this was what our father would have wanted. His words comforted us, because "pulling the plug" probably always creates some guilt for those making such decisions.

My father was a fine man. Practically on his own, he supported himself through college, thereafter securing a fine job with a utility company lasting for 40 years, climbing the ranks to assistant division manager. He provided for the family, and provided well. I still remember him buying one of the first Bendix washing machines for Mother. Bolted tightly to the kitchen floor, it seemed the whole house shook during the spin cycle. He became a 32nd degree Mason, an officer in Kiwanis, and a respected member of the Lutheran Church.

He was honorable, admired, always responsible, and a dapper dresser. Toward the end of his life, countless people at the retirement home expressed their esteem and love for him. Even his favorite restaurant waitress sent flowers for the memorial service.

However, I wish we could have explored the principle of opposites and what Todd Pearson describes as "cultural shadow." We both share a European ancestry, Dad being third generation American and I being a fourth removed from our German heritage. After an unfortunate incident during a visit several months before he died, he confessed having a temper, inherited from his father.

Lon Hatfield speaks about family constellations and behaviors passed along from generation to generation. Both my father and I are linked through to a very harmful belief system. As described by Alice Miller in her book, *For Your Own Good*, in essence it deems that humans are essentially bad and, given an opportunity, they will get worse. Therefore, "Children must be 'broken' as soon as possible."[1] Early beatings to 'get the hell out' of children may result in conforming, responsible, and highly structured behaviors as we grow into adulthood. However, the ensuing repressed anger often erupts into the violence we witness so often in our culture today.

Such destructive perceptions and experiences are apparently widespread in several heritages and infect the medical profession as well. Martin Doot reported his belief that 80% to 90% of physician outbursts of anger spring from early childhood experiences.

I wish my father and I could have discussed and liberated ourselves from this concealed history of abuse. We both need to forgive our fathers and our father's fathers. Failing to do so as individuals and as cultures, we are doomed to continue these inherited constellations and harmful emotional expressions.

In any case, some contemporary theoretical physicists suggest that we do not live in a universe, but in a multiverse of many dimensions where time is more circular than linear. If so, as spooky as it seems, my father may in fact be reading these reflections and healing in his own way. In any case, sharing such stories as mine is one of the many strategies available to people contributing to such healing.

---

[1] Miller, A. *For Your Own Good: Hidden Cruelty in Child-Rearing and the Roots of Violence.* 3rd ed. New York, NY: Noonday Press; 1990: 59.

Linda's Concluding Reflections

Our stories become a gift we give each other. Perhaps Jeffery Roth said it better when he noted, "When I am telling my story it is a form of prayer, and when I am learning something from other people I experience it as a meditative event."

As such, writing this book was an incredible gift. We feel deeply grateful to those who participated and are honored by their trust in sharing even a little of their stories. We hope we have kept that trust. Each visit and conversation offered us more than we could possibly have expected. In many cases, their stories moved us to tears.

Arguably, this book is slightly skewed in that it reflects only those physicians who agreed to be interviewed and who had interest in talking about their own stories and their perceptions of soul. We do believe, however, that their thoughts and personal journeys have important implications to others. We offer the book in the hope that people will come to understand the remarkable gifts and passion physicians bring to their calling. If, by sharing their stories, this book inspires others in their journey toward medicine, or if it rekindles the passion and joy of medicine for others, then we have shared something of enormous value.

At the end of any work, it is tempting to summarize a set of particular findings, or the *takeaways*, as some might define them. Stories, by their very nature, are not linear sets of itemized results. Instead, they reflect individuals' particular journeys, their challenges, joys, sorrows, and hopes. Given that, however, it is amazing, the similar themes we found running through many of these stories, regardless of the physician's age, background, specialty, or length of career.

First, it is the passion. Most of the physicians with whom we spoke view medicine as a joy, their passion and calling. In some cases, practicing medicine is literally something that they "cannot not do," a profession filled with wonder and mystery. We are reminded of Joseph Campbell's words referring to being led by unseen hands. Medicine is a sacred journey for some, one that is shared for a time by physician and patient, at least temporarily. Some describe such a shared journey as a gift from God, an honor, and privilege. In a number of instances, physicians came into their particular medical passion almost through happenstance. We are particularly reminded of the stories of Tom Cornwell and Martin Doot.

In so many cases, life skills of caring and compassion for others were at the heart of their work, even in the midst of personal adversity. Often the important messages learned from their parents or from mentors form the foundation of their beliefs. For example, Ron Williams states, "What makes me stand out is what my mother taught me about relating to people before I reached the age of 5. She taught us the Golden Rule, to be polite and respectful of other people. Through such basic instruction, we learned to be sensitive to the situations of people."

If there is a central theme of being a good physician, it is that of really connecting with another. It is that which motivates even the new, young physicians like Maile Anslinger and Emily Transue.

Connecting to something outside oneself, whether identified as *soul* or related to spirituality, is woven throughout many of the stories. As Roy Farrell said, "I believe that, in the final analysis, every interaction is spiritual in nature—as is every calling and every career—but in medicine the spiritual connection is so much closer to the surface. This spiritual connection is a great part of the inherent reward I get from being a physician. It involves touching the whole person in ways that are special and privileged. In this respect, hopefully the doctor–patient relationship is rewarding to both of us."

Then, too, many physicians acknowledged the important role prayer plays in the delivery of care and in the healing process.

Not surprisingly, the changing health care environment is a topic of much concern. Being resilient in such chaotic times is critical to continuing to practice with the same high level of enthusiasm that was present in the beginning of their practices. Sharing one's story, offering mutual support, and having a faith system are among the key components of being resilient. Resiliency enables physicians to reconnect with their passion. Although a number of the physicians we interviewed admitted some degree of pessimism, most were optimistic and hopeful about the future of medicine. In the beginning of this book, we said that, ultimately, this was a book about hope. Although personally hopeful about medicine at the outset, we are even more hopeful after hearing these stories.

For both of us, it is exciting to hear physicians speak about their mission in these terms and to provide an arena such as this book so others can hear about it also. Listening to physicians' stories is a simple, yet profound way to grasp their souls. It is unfortunate that sometimes patients are not privy to such accounts. It requires some willingness to be vulnerable, but we believe knowing something of each other's personal story greatly enhances the unique healing partnership between patient and physician. As Sanjev Parikh said so well,

> "If we can rekindle the soul of the physician, then he or she will be able to look at these problems from a different perspective and will not let them affect the core of the doctor–patient relationship."

Having read these stories, we invite you, our reader, to share your own story. Physicians often confess that they typically do not share their stories with other colleagues or even their practice partners, sometimes not even with their spouses. We hope to provide a way that physicians can begin to share such journeys with others. Understanding the power and importance of storytelling, the AMA created a secure opportunity for physicians to begin sharing their stories by creating a new forum link on their Web site. This Internet venue allows physicians to connect in dialogue. It also will offer information and resources for enhancing soul in medicine. There are other ways of creating opportunities to introduce personal story sharing. A number of these resources are listed in the next section. We are also interested in hearing from our readers. Our e-mail address is jlhenry@aol.com.

There is no better way to conclude this book than by inviting you to share your own personal story and ongoing journey. Now, begin. We wish you well.

Strategies for Caring for Oneself

Share Your Story

As hopefully demonstrated throughout this book, sharing one's story with others who will listen with empathy and without judgment serves as a significant way to heal and to grow as a person. Stories preserve our life experiences and often more deeply and meaningfully connect us to others. Storytelling also becomes a channel connecting us to soul and spirit.

In advance of our interview, we sent a list of questions to each physician. A number of physicians spoke about how helpful it was, in general, to reflect upon them. They saw it as a way to step back in time from a busy practice to evaluate their purpose and passion for the profession. We encourage you to do the same and to share your thoughts with others. Here is a list of some of the questions we asked:

- What early experiences led you to medicine as a vocation?
- What are you passionate about in your work?
- Describe a situation in your work when you experienced wonder and mystery.
- What does the word *soul* mean to you?
- Describe the characteristics of a physician who is connected to soul/spirit.
- What are some ways a physician can take care of himself or herself emotionally and spiritually?
- In what nonclinical ways do you develop yourself as a person? What do you read?
- How do you enhance a sense of community in your life?
- How have you dealt with a mistake you made?
- Describe a setback in your career and how you responded to it?
- Can you share a humorous event in your practice?
- Are you optimistic or pessimistic about the future of medicine?
- At your memorial service after you die, what would you hope your patients would say about you as a tribute?
- Who are your heroes?

Why not approach some of your colleagues, inviting them to meet periodically for an hour or two to reflect on such questions as a group? We suggest it will significantly deepen your sense of medical community. Sharing stories with other doctors serves to connect and enhance the joy of medicine. We propose the following guidelines for such a gathering:

1. Each person pledges strict confidentiality. No story may be shared outside the group without that person's permission.
2. Privacy must be honored. Each participant determines information to be shared or not shared.
3. People may choose to pass when sharing stories about a particular topic.
4. Participants commit to not interrupt each other or dominate the group's time together.
5. Speak in the "first person." ("I think," I feel,")
6. Acknowledge that each person's story is an interpretation. A person's perception will not be reinterpreted or contradicted.
7. Agree not to turn the session into a "pity party" of complaints about the current health care environment.
8. Commit to a specific schedule and set time parameters. For example, the group might meet twice a month for a period of 3 months, then evaluate whether you wish to continue.

Live with Forward-focused Questions

In *Letters to a Young Poet*, Rainer Maria Rilke states,

". . . try to love *the questions themselves* as if they were locked rooms or books written in a very foreign language. Don't search for the answers, which could not be given to you now, because you would not be able to live them. And the point is, to live everything. *Live* the questions now. Perhaps then, someday far in the future, you will gradually, without even noticing it, live your way into the answer."[1]

Living forward-moving questions involves allowing the answers to come to you. It engages not a passive approach to life, but an active-receptive stance. For example, you might ask, "How am I to live the rest of my life? What is my destiny or calling?" We remain active

---

[1] Rilke RM. *Letters to a Young Poet*. New York, NY: W.W. Norton & Co; 1994.

during the ensuing days and weeks, but open to guidance from inner and outer voices of wisdom.

In terms of the process of forgiveness, this approach suggests utilizing the experience and energy of past wounds to refocus on the future. If you have been violated, how can you prevent its reoccurrence in your life and to others? It's the Mothers Against Drunk Driving method.

Practice the Process of Forgiveness[2]

Earlier in this book, Janis Bridge mentioned the importance of forgiveness, especially the role it plays in the Jewish ritual called The Day of Atonement. Don Greggain spoke about how difficult it was for his mother to forgive the attending physician during the death of her child. Wayne Day addressed the problems associated with making a medical mistake and his belief that honesty is the best policy; unless there has been major damage, people are usually willing to forgive.

In his book, *Healing the Wounds, A Physician Looks at His Work,* David Hilfiker points out that through forgiveness, we become better people. For these reasons, and because we believe it is vital to both physical and emotional healing, we wish to include some perceptions about how the process of forgiveness works. While one word "forgiveness" is not particulary limited to religious traditions, in the Old Testament, the translation from the Latin means basically "to lift," while in the New Testiment, it means "to send away."

Each day, newspapers and newscasts report events of brutality. They surface in many forms: physical, emotional, social, sexual, political, financial, vocational, and even religious abuse. Though we may deny it, rarely in our society can we come across a person who has not been traumatized in one way or another.

Like physical healing, forgiveness is a process. In particular, Harry Chinchinian underscored the relationships between mind, emotion, and the immune system. Although it takes time and cannot be forced by giving lip service to it, to forgive undoubtedly contributes to physical well-being.

---

[2] We are indebted to The Rev Dr Kathlyn James, senior pastor of First United Methodist Church, Seattle, Washington, for much of this content.

In their book, *Forgiveness: How to Make Peace With Your Past and Get on With Life*, Sidney and Suzanne Simon list five stages involved in the process of forgiveness. They also offer a host of strategies to successfully move through the stages to a time of hope and healing.[3] Brief descriptions of the stages follow:

Claiming the Pain. The first stage in the process, claiming the pain, stands opposite to denial. Bob Barnes spoke about how, for many years, he denied the reality and pain associated with his father's suicide. Both Lynn Hankes and Gary Olbrich denied their problems with alcohol before starting on the road to recovery. Denial happens especially when pain is new and deep, just as shock becomes the natural reaction when we experience a physical injury.

Claiming the pain requires hard work, especially if it contradicts "public evidence,"—by this we mean the mask we wear, the persona or "Sunday self." This might be why some physicians face a difficult time accepting themselves as wounded healers, because the wounded self can remain hidden in the shadows of one's personality. We hope that some of the testimonies in this book will stimulate those in denial to move beyond it, to claim and express the pain.

Claiming the hurt often necessitates hard work. No one really wants to claim something painful. Courage is required to let yourself remember, resurrect, and appreciate the gravity of a hurt inflicted on you, but this first stage of forgiveness cannot be bypassed. We must recognize the extent of our injuries.

Self-blame. The second stage involves ridding oneself of self-blame. In their book, *Creativity in Business*, Michael Ray and Rochelle Myers, coin the phrase, The Voice of Judgment (VOJ).[4] It inflicts us with serious wounds, in some instances accusing us of causing the abuse inflicted upon ourselves. We might say, "Something I said or did must have caused the harm done to me. "Am I that bad a person that I was beat with a paddle?" The VOJ often imposes upon us inappropriate and harmful "shoulds" and "oughts." For example, someone is told, "I know you were attacked, but you should have stayed off the streets at night." Or, "If you know what's good for you, you ought to keep your mouth shut."

---

[3] Simon, Simons, *Forgiveness*. New York, NY: Warner Books; 1991.

[4] Ray M, Myers R. *Creativity in Business*. New York, NY: Doubleday; 1989.

Because they often must deal with life-threatening illnesses, we suspect that physicians especially fall victim to the VOJ. "Did I make the wrong diagnosis? Was the treatment appropriate?"

Moving away from self-blame requires a great deal of gentleness toward oneself. Todd Pearson shared with us the importance of self-compassion. Professional caregivers need to be as caring for themselves as they are for others. Janis Bridge takes mini-vacations as one solution to quelling the VOJ.

"You are not responsible for the rain that falls, but only for your reaction to it."

— Virginia Satir
Self Esteem (1975)

Letting go of victimhood. This third stage of forgiveness involves acknowledging that we have been hurt, unjustly so, and it was not our fault. The problem comes when we begin to wallow in self-pity, lashing out at innocent bystanders and going through life expecting the worst. When this happens, we sink into a mire of helplessness and hopelessness. "Victim" becomes not just what happened to us, but *who we think we are.*

We all know people who are stuck at this stage. Most of us have been there ourselves a time or two. Relating it specifically to the advent of managed care, Richard Payne speaks about physicians attending a "pity party," commiserating over the loss of the golden years of medicine. It puts us into a vicious cycle. First, someone harms us. Then we blame ourselves for its occurrence. The conclusion is we are worthless. So we go around setting ourselves up to be harmed again.

One way to leave the pity party is to attend a compassion party. It involves joining a support group where we discover our hurts are not unique. We learn that there are people moving on with their lives, refusing to join the pity party.

Unloading anger. The fourth stage in the forgiveness process requires us to appropriately unload our anger. Refusing to join a pity party and become a part of the vicious cycle of martyrdom, we say, "I won't put up with it anymore. I'm taking action!"

When expressed in a timely and fitting manner, anger serves as a powerful, positive force. There is a "Peanuts" cartoon in which Linus stands on the beach with a pile of rocks next to him. He hurls one stone at a time into the water, saying, "This is for wife beaters, this is for hungry children, this is for drunk drivers." Such rituals are vital to our healing.

In health care, the organization Physicians for Social Responsibility, serves as a more visible example of suitable indignation. In addition, Janis Bridge reports, "My most recent tirade, and I'm thinking about writing an article about this, involves physician abandonment." Her anger about managed care forcing patients to change physicians finds expression through her writing about it. And, frustrated by the physical abuse he witnesses in the emergency department, Roy Farrell participated in initiating a program called *Cops and Docs*, teaching junior high school students about the medical and legal consequences of using guns.

Integration/resilience. The last stage of the forgiveness process is called integration. It involves resilience and the ability to move forward. It represents the final destination of the journey, the reason we are willing to embark on it in the first place. At this stage, we recognize that, although we were indeed hurt, we did, in fact, survive. Our painful past experiences took something from us and gave us things as well. We finally put the past in its proper perspective, neither dwelling on it nor forgetting it. We see it for what it is—a part of who we are, but not all of who we are today or who we can be in the future. There emerges a sense of moving forward. Like a wounded bird that heals and flies again, the hard-won freedom of forgiveness is ours. As the adage goes, "Today is the first day of the rest of your life."

> "Human pain does not let go of its grip at one point in time. Rather it works its way out of our consciousness over time. There is a season of sadness. A season of anger. A season of tranquility. A season of hope. . . ."
>
> — Robert Veninga
> *Gift of Hope* (1985)

Even if the person(s) who has harmed us is not sorry, or if they have died, the power of the harming event is released. We become free to make our own choices to live and love again. We may even contemplate the possibility of rebuilding our relationship with harming parties. At the very least, we begin to view them as having been wounded themselves by life events. However, we don't have to "work things out" unless we desire to and if the other person is open to change and reconciliation. In any case, freedom involves expanding and embracing your options.

For physicians, arriving at this stage may be like reconnecting to one's passion for medicine or finding a new direction for that passion. For example, Gary Olbrich declares "My vocational passion is trying to prevent some of the tragedies that occurred in my life from happening to other physicians." Joy Kim announces, "Today I am more of a wounded healer. By learning about what this concretely means, I can offer so much more to people." Faced with the possibility of having to close his practice because of managed care, Wayne Day expands his options, reporting, "Right now I am already refocusing my energy by engaging in medical mission activities." A recovering workaholic, Jeffrey Roth declares, "For me, having boundaries around my work is very important. I have many activities in my life that are not work. Being in intimate personal relationships is very necessary. I have hobbies and interests, but what is vital is how they help me to experience my aliveness. For example, I like to roller blade."

Pray

A significant number of physicians interviewed for this book shared, as appropriate, that they either pray for or with some of their patients. We approach this subject in the broadest sense, as described by Ann and Barry Ulanov in their book, *Primary Speech.* At the time of publication, Ann was a professor at Union Seminary in New York and Barry a professor of English at Barnard College. They assert that, whether conscious of it or not, everyone prays, whether they know it or call it prayer. It is elemental discourse, such as pondering, "Why I am here?" To pray is to seek wisdom and guidance.

> "We pray every time we ask for help, understanding, or strength, in or out of religion. . . . Our movements, stillness, the expressions on our faces, our tone of voice, our actions, what we dream and daydream, as well as what we actually put into words say who and what we are."[5]

As such, there is no best way to pray or correct words to use. However, in his book, *Healing Words,* Larry Dossey, MD, suggests that a nondirective approach may be most suitable.[6] Here, we do not petition an outcome, such as telling God or the universe what to do. For example, as appropriate during career guidance sessions, Jim may suggest the following: "God (or your own metaphor), as you know, I am unhappy in my current job. I would like some guidance and I am promising in advance to pay attention." The latter "paying attention" refers to the active-receptive stance we men-

---

[5] Ulanov A, Ulanov B. *Primary Speech.* Atlanta, GA: John Knox Press; 1982, 1.
[6] Dossey, L. *Healing Words.* New York, NY: HarperCollins; 1993.

tioned earlier. One might actively seek more satisfying work but be open to surprise and unexpected developments.

In a health care situation, a suggested stance might be to simply imagine a patient being surrounded by a shield of light. Or, one might pray, "Your will be done." As several physicians mentioned, death is not necessarily a tragedy but can be an answer to healing. In light of her experience surrounding her daughter's cancer, Nancy Neubauer in particular learned how to graciously live in the precious present.

Express Gratitude

According to research conducted by Robert A. Emmons at the University of California, practicing the art of gratitude makes you healthier, smarter, and more energetic.[7] Emmons made participants in his study keep weekly journals of gratitude and then compared them with others who didn't jot down who they should thank and what for. The grateful ones, he found, "exercised more regularly, reported fewer physical symptoms, felt better about their lives as a whole, and where more optimistic about the upcoming week."

In the final analysis, gratitude is a measure of how alive we are, for life itself is a gift. The universe is a gift.

"The universe may
Be as great as they say.
But it wouldn't be missed
If it didn't exist."

— Piet Hein

[7] Gratitude makes you healthier, smarter, [NewsMax.com Web site]. Avaiable at http://www.newsmax.com. Accessed January 10, 2001.

BIBLIOGRAPHY

Campbell J. *The Power of Myth*. New York, NY: Doubleday; 1988.

Carlson R, Shield B. *Healers on Healing*. Los Angeles, CA: Tarcher; 1989.

Cleaveland C. *Sacred Space*. Philadelphia, PA: American College of Physicians; 1998.

Cole RL. *The Gentle Greeting*. Naperville, IL: Sourcebooks; 1998.

Dossey L. *Reinventing Medicine*. San Francisco, CA: HarperSanFrancisco; 1999.

Fischer-Williams M. *Emotions of a Physician, Discovering the Needs of Doctors to Understand Their Own Experiences*. Milwaukee, WI: Gearhart-Edwards Press; 1993.

Gerber L. *Married to Their Careers*. New York, NY: Tavistock Publications; 1983.

Guggenbühl-Craig A. *Power in the Helping Professions*. Irving, TX: Spring Publications; 1979.

Hilfiker D. *Healing the Wounds, A Physician Looks at His Work*. New York, NY: Penguin Books, Viking Penguin, Inc.; 1987.

Hutschnecker A. *The Will to Live*. New York, NY: Cornerstone Library; 1978.

Jaworski J. *Synchronicity: The Inner Path of Leadership*. San Francisco, CA: Berrett-Koehler; 1996.

Koenig H. *The Healing Power of Faith*. New York, NY: Simon & Schuster; 1999.

Levoy G. *Callings*. New York, NY: Harmony Books; 1997.

Lowenstein J. *The Midnight Meal and Other Essays About Doctors, Patients and Medicine*. New Haven, CN: Yale University; 1997.

Lown B. *The Lost Art of Healing*. Boston, MA: Houghton Mifflin Company; 1996.

Loxterkamp D. *A Measure of My Days, The Journal of a Country Doctor*. Hanover, NH: University Press of New England; 1997.

Magee M, D'Antonio M. *The Best Medicine, Doctors, Patients, and the Covenant of Caring*. New York, NY: St. Martin's Press; 1999.

Mandell H, Spiro H, eds. *When Doctors Get Sick*. New York, NY: Plenum Medical Book Co.; 1987.

Marion R. *Learning to Play God, The Coming of Age of a Young Doctor*. Reading, MA: Addison-Wesley; 1991.

Needleman J. *The Way of the Physician*. San Francisco, CA: Harper & Row; 1985.

Needleman J. *Time and the Soul: Where Has All the Meaningful Time Gone?...and How to Get It Back.* New York, NY: Currency/Doubleday; 1998.

Nuland S. *How We Die.* New York, NY: Alfred A. Knopf; 1993.

Nuland S. *The Mysteries Within.* New York, NY: Simon & Schuster; 2000.

Osler W. *Aequanimitas.* Philadelphia, PA: The Blakiston Company; 1932.

Palmer PJ. *Let Your Life Speak, Listening for the Voice of Vocation.* San Francisco, CA: Jossey-Bass; 1999.

PBS Video, *Medicine at the Crossroads.* New York, NY: Thirteen/WNET; 1993.

Remen RN. *The Human Patient.* Garden City, NY: Anchor Press; 1980.

Remen RN. *Kitchen Table Wisdom.* New York, NY: Riverhead Books; 1996.

Stone R. *The Healing Art of Storytelling.* New York, NY: Hyperion; 1996.

Sulmasy DP. *The Healer's Calling.* New York, NY: Paulist Press; 1997.

Thomas L. *The Youngest Science, Notes of a Medicine-Watcher.* New York, NY: Viking Press; 1983.